# A Practical Book of Pharmacology

**Dr. Rajshree Dahiya**
Assistant Professor
Jai Narain Vyas University
Jodhpur - 342001 (Rajasthan)

SCIENTIFIC®
PUBLISHERS
New Delhi • Jodhpur

SCIENTIFIC®
PUBLISHERS
New Delhi • Jodhpur

*Published by:*

**Jodhpur**
5 A, New Pali Road, P.O. Box 91 Jodhpur - 342 001 Rajasthan (India)
E-mail: info@scientificpub.com
Website:
www.scientificpubonline.com

**New Delhi**
4806/24, Ansari Road, Daryaganj,
New Delhi - 110 002 (India)



ISBN: 978-81-96247-11-9 (HB)
eISBN: 978-81-962471-3-3

Printed in India

# Table of Contents

# Pharmacology-I
## (Semester-IV)

# Experiment No. 1

## Object: Introduction to experimental pharmacology.

## Introduction:

Pharmacology is the science which deals with the study of drugs. The word 'PHARMACOLOGY' is derived from the Greek words '*Pharmakon*' (a drug or poison) and *logos* (discourse). It deals with interaction of exogenously administered chemical molecules (drug) with living system. It broadly covers the information about the history, source, physicochemical properties, physiological properties, mechanism of action, absorption, distribution, metabolism and excretion of drugs. Drugs are chemical agents used for the purpose of diagnosis, prevention relief or cure of a disease in man or animals. The word drug is derived from the French word 'drogue' meaning herb.

Pharmacology as an experimental science was ushered by Rudolf Buchheim who founded the first institute of pharmacology in 1847 in Germany. In the later part of the $19^{th}$ century, Oswald Schmiedeberg, regarded as the 'Father of pharmacology', together with his many disciples like J Langley, T Frazer, P Ehrlich, AJ Clark, JJ Abel propounded some of the fundamental concepts in pharmacology.

The two main divisions of pharmacology are pharmacodynamics and pharmacokinetics.

**Pharmacodynamics:** The pharmacodynamics term comes from greek word: dynamics-power. It the study of drug effects, which includes physiological and biochemical effects of drugs and their mechanism of action at any organ/system, such as adrenaline beta-1receptors in heart, that is a G-protein coupled receptor, which stimulates adenyl cyclase and increase intracellular cAMP which leads top cardiac stimulation.

**Pharmacokinetics:** The pharmacokinetics term comes from greek word: kinesis-movement. Pharmacokinetics is movement of drug in and alteration of drugs by the body. It is the qualitative study of drug movement which includes absorption, distribution, metabolism and excretion (ADME) of the drug. E.g. paracetamol is rapidly and almost completely absorbed orally attaining peak blood levels at 30-60 min; 25% bound to plasma proteins, widely and almost uniformly distributed in the body; extensively metabolized in the liver, primary by glucuronide and sulfate conjugation into inactive metabolites which are excreted in urine; has a plasma half life of 2-3 hours and a clearance value of 5ml/kg/min.

## Some other important aspects of pharmacology are:

**Pharmacotherapeutics:** It is the application of pharmacological information together with knowledge of the disease for its prevention, mitigation or cure.

**Clinical pharmacology:** The branch concerned with the scientific studies on the effects of drug treatment in human being.

**Chemotherapy:** It is the treatment of systemic infection/malignancy with specific drugs that have selective toxicity for the infecting organism/malignant cell with no/minimal effects on the host cells.

**Pharmacy:** It is the art and science of compounding and dispensing drugs or preparing suitable dosage forms for administration of drugs to man or animals.

**Toxicology:** It is the study of poisonous effect of drugs and other chemicals (household, environmental pollutant, industrial, agricultural, homicidal) with emphasis on detection, prevention and treatment of poisonings.

**Pharmacoepidemiology:** Study of effects of drugs in large numbers of people.

**Pharmacogenomics:** Application of genomic technologies to new drug discovery and further characterization of older drugs.

**Neuropharmacology:** Effects of medication on central and peripheral nervous system functioning.

**Psychopharmacology:** Effects of medication on the psyche; observing changed behaviors of the body and mind, and how molecular events are manifested in a measurable behavioral form.

**Pharmacogenetics:** Clinical testing of genetic variation that gives rise to differing response to drugs.

**Theoretical Pharmacology:** Study of metrics in pharmacology.

**Posology:** How medicines are dosed. It also depends upon various factors like age, climate, weight, sex, and so on.

**Pharmacovigilance (PV)**: It is defined as the science and activities relating to the detection, assessment, understanding and prevention of adverse effects or any other drug-related problem.

**Side effects:** A secondary but predictable effect, typically undesirable effect of a drug or medical treatment.

**Adverse effects:** A secondary but unpredictable effect, typically undesirable effect of a drug or medical treatment.

**Toxic effects:** Harmful effects of the drug which is related to dose (Excess).

Experimental pharmacology is relatively the youngest branch of basic medical sciences. The advancement in the field of electrophysiology, biochemistry, and molecular biology and electronic or digital recording systems and softwares have enriched and broadened the horizons of experimental pharmacology.

## Objectives of the experimental pharmacology:

- To screen drug substance for their biological activities.
- To study the toxicity of drugs.
- To study mechanism of action and site of action of the drug.

## Experimental Pharmacology involves:

### a. Preclinical Experiments:

- Which consist of animal studies for deciding the safety, efficacy, pharmacokinetics and pharmacodynamics of a new drug or a new drug formulation.
- The purpose of pre-clinical study is to develop adequate data to decide that it is reasonably safe to proceed with human trials of the drug.
- Experiments are generally performed on rodent like mouse, rat, guinea pig, hamster, rabbit.
- After successful result, experiments are performed on larger animals like cat, dog, monkey.
- As the evaluation progresses unfavorable compounds get rejected at each step.
- So, that only few out of thousands reach the stage when administration to man is considered.

### b. Clinical Experiments:

These follow preclinical studies. In clinical pharmacology, efficacy, safety, and pharmacokinetics of a drug substance is determined through its use in healthy human volunteers and patient populations under controlled conditions. Only those drugs which are found safe and effective in preclinical (animal) studies are further investigated in such studies.

## Phases of Clinical Trial:

**Phase I:** First in man - safety

This trial is on the 20-80 numbers of healthy volunteers. In this the safety of drug, tolerability, pharmacokinetics and side effects is studied.

**Phase II:** First in patient - dose, dosage form

This trial is on 100-300 numbers of patients as well as healthy volunteers. This study is carried out for efficacy and dosage along with toxicology study.

**Phase III:** Efficacy, ADRs

These trials are carried out in large patients ranging from 800-3000 patients. This consists the study of comparing the new drug with existing drugs.

**Phase IV** or Post marketing surveillance: Evaluation in the real clinical setting

Post marketing surveillance in patients for detecting any rare or long term adverse drug reactions.

## Pharmacologists and their achievements:

| S.No. | Name of scientists | Achievements |
|---|---|---|
| 1. | Oswald schmiedeberg | Father of Pharmacology |
| 2. | Rudolf Buchheim | Pioneer of experimental pharmacology |
| 3. | John Jacob abel | Father of American Pharmacology |
| 4. | Louis Lasagna | Father of clinical pharmacology |
| 5. | Francois magendie | Pioneer of experimental physiology |
| 6. | Claude Bernard | Father of physiology |
| 7. | Paul Ehrlich | Father of chemotherapy |
| 8. | Sir Ram Nath Chopra | Father of Indian pharmacology |

## VIVA-VOCE

**Q.1 Explain different phases of clinical trial.**

**Ans: Phase I:** First in man - safety

This trial is on the 20-80 numbers of healthy volunteers. In this the safety of drug, tolerability, pharmacokinetics and side effects is studied.

**Phase II:** First in patient - dose, dosage form

This trial is on 100-300 numbers of patients as well as healthy volunteers. This study carried out for efficacy and dosage along with toxicology study.

**Phase III:** Efficacy, ADRs

These trials carried out in large patients ranging from 800-3000 patients. This consist the study of comparing the new drug with existing drugs.

**Phase IV or Post marketing surveillance:** Evaluation in the real clinical setting

Post marketing surveillance in patients for detecting any rare or long term adverse drug reactions.

**Q.2 Give objectives of experimental pharmacology.**

**Ans:** Objectives of the experimental pharmacology:

- To screen drug substance for their biological activities.
- To study the toxicity of drugs.
- To study mechanism of action and site of action of the drug.

**Q.3 Explain in detail about pre-clinical study.**

**Ans:** Pre-clinical study contains in-vivo and in-vitro experiments which consist of animal studies for deciding the safety, efficacy, pharmacokinetics and pharmacodynamics of a new drug or a new drug formulation. The purpose of pre-clinical study is to develop adequate data to decide that it is reasonably safe to proceed with human trials of the drug. Experiments are generally performed on rodent like mouse, rat, guinea pig, hamster, rabbit. After successful result, experiments are performed on larger animals like cat, dog, monkey. As the evaluation progresses unfavorable compounds get rejected at each step. So, that only few out of thousands reach the stage when administration to man is considered.

**Q.4 Define pharmacology.**

**Ans:** Pharmacology is the science which deals with the study of drugs. the word 'PHARMACOLOGY' is derived from the Greek words *'Pharmakon'* (a drug or poison) and *logos* (discourse). It deals with interaction of exogenously administered chemical molecules (drug) with living system.

**Q.5 Define drugs.**

**Ans:** Drugs are chemical agents used for the purpose of diagnosis, prevention, relief or cure of a disease in man or animals. The word drug is derived from the French word 'drogue' meaning herb.

# Experiment No. 2

## Object: To study commonly used Instruments in experimental pharmacology.

### 1. Instruments used for experiments using isolated tissue preparation:

**Sherrington recording drum and student's organ bath:** Sherrington recording drum and student's organ bath assembly for intestine was first designed by Rudolph Magnus in 1904. Many of the institutions and research laboratories use the smoke paper or ink pen on white paper for recording the tissue response.

**Sherrington Recording Drum (Using Kymograph):** It is the instrument on which physiological responses such as contraction and relaxation of a muscle are recorded. It consists of a *heavy base* and a vertical *shaft*. Heavy base gives stability to drum. It has;

i. **Base hoofs** (legs) with adjustable leveling screws to keep drum horizontal if surface of the table is uneven.
ii. **Side hoof** to turn the drum on its side so that shaft becomes horizontal.
iii. **Gear rod** arrangement with fast, slow and neutral gears and clutch (starter). The gear rod is attached to a cone wheel which has 4 pulley grooves. Desirable speed of drum can be obtained by changing gear position and shaft drum pulley connections.
iv. **Contact screw** on the surface. A wire can be fixed from main plug to convey the current through base.
v. **Contact foil** with a contact screw mounted on an insulated material on the superior surface of the base. Second wire can be connected here.
vi. **Drum cylinder** is a brass or iron cylinder around which a paper is wrapped and smoked. Drum with smoked paper is fitted on vertical shaft. At the base of vertical shaft, there are two projecting strikers which can be drawn apart to set any desired angle between them. When the striker makes contact with foil, the circuit occurs.

These days electrical drum is more commonly used. This is similar to Sherrington recording drum but speed is controlled electrically with the help of gear.

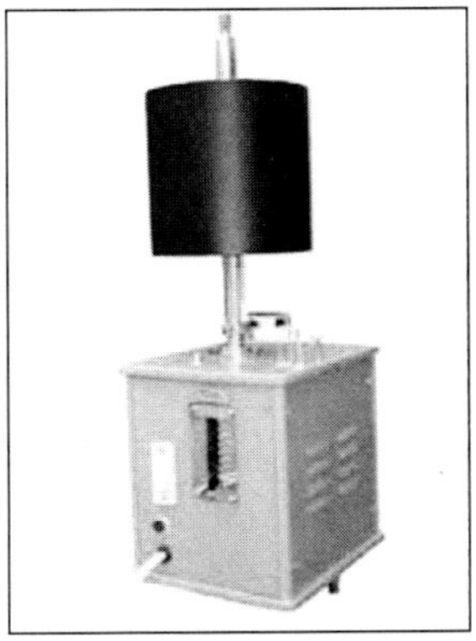

**Sherrington Drum**

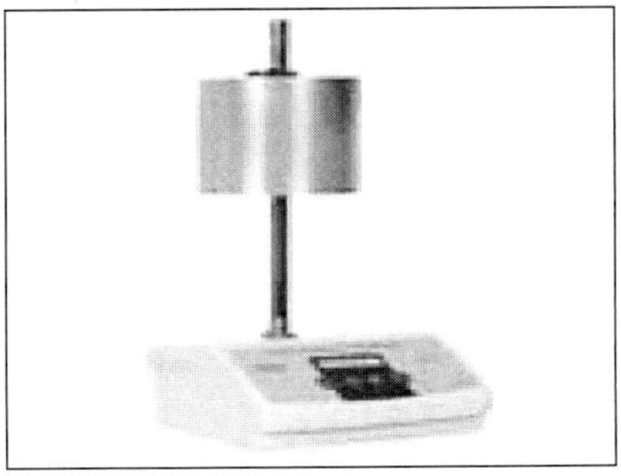

**Electrical drum**

**Student's organ bath:** The tissue bath used to put the animal tissue for studying the drug actions is called student organ bath.

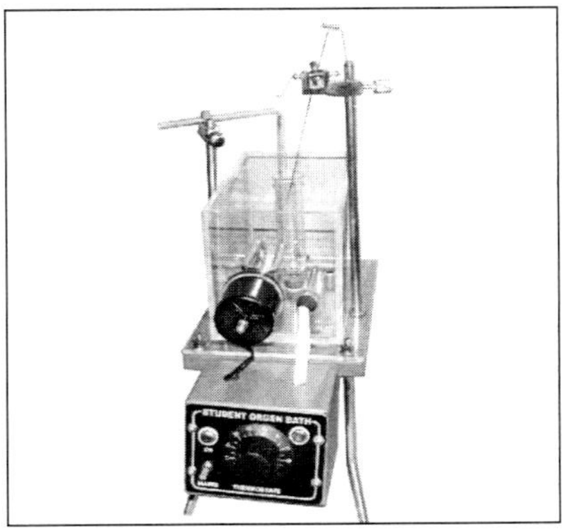


**Student's organ bath**

## The organ bath essentially consists of:

i. **An outer jacket** made up of steel or glass or Perspex.
ii. **The inner organ or tissue bath** made up of glass with a capacity varying from 10 -50 ml.
iii. **Thermostatically** controlled heating rod.
iv. **Stirrer** to keep water in the outer jacket at uniform temperature.
v. **Oxygen or delivery glass tube** which also serves as tissue holder.
vi. **A reservoir** contains the physiological salt solution.
vii. **Glass coil:** one end of which is connected to the physiological salt solution.
viii. **Meriotte bottle** is used to record or keep the physiological solution used in the experimental. It should be periodically cleaned with HCl and chromic acid. It is named after French physiologist Edme Mariotte.
ix. **The student organ bath** having two units of inner tissue bath is called double unit organ bath.
x. **Recording lever**: This is used to record the contractions or relaxations of the isolated tissue preparation. The writing levers are light in weight, rigid and are generally made up of wood, light aluminium or stainless steel.

**Parts of lever**:

a. Effort arm: Point where force is to be applied
b. Load arm: Effect observed due to application of force.

## Types of lever:

**I. Isotonic type:**

Change in length due to contraction is recorded while the tension on the muscle remains the same. Examples of isotonic levers are simple lever, frontal writing lever.

**II. Isometric type:**

Isometric recording measures increase in tension of the tissue when the length of the tissue is kept constant.

## The common recording levers used in the laboratory are:

A. **Simple lever (side-way writing):** It is the simplest type of lever made up of wood, stainless steel or aluminium. A celluloid writing tip (stylus) is attached at the end of the longer arm. The contractions are recorded as curved lines.
B. **Frontal writing lever (writes frontally):** This lever is designed in such a way that the writing point rotates freely about its axle. This helps in reducing the tension between the smoked paper and the recording tip. The contractions are recorded as straight line.

C. **Starling's heart lever:** This lever is used to record the contraction of the heart. The difference between this and other isotonic levers is that the fulcrum lies at one end beyond the point of attachment.

D. **Brodie's universal lever:** It is a general utility lever having axis screwed with two nuts between which the interchangeable levers are clamped.

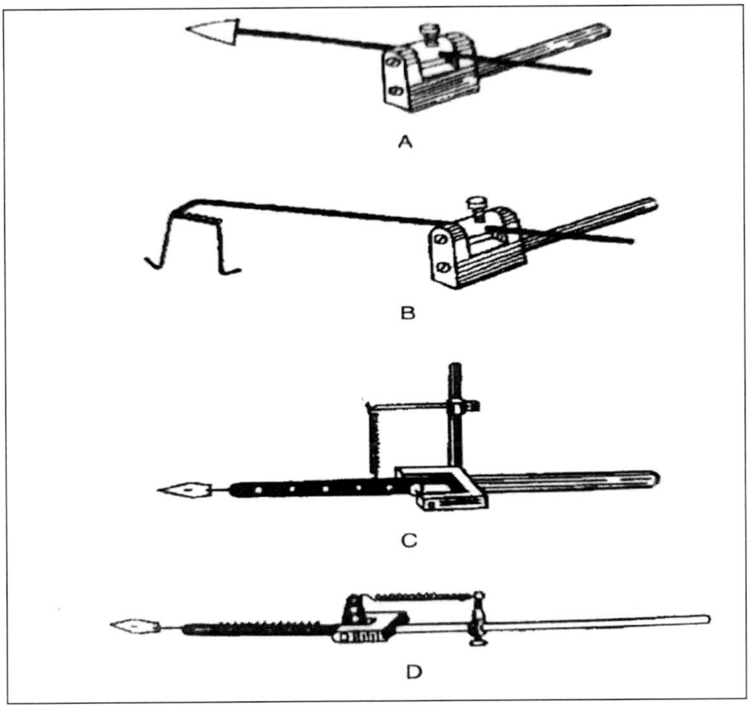


## 2. Rotarod Apparatus:

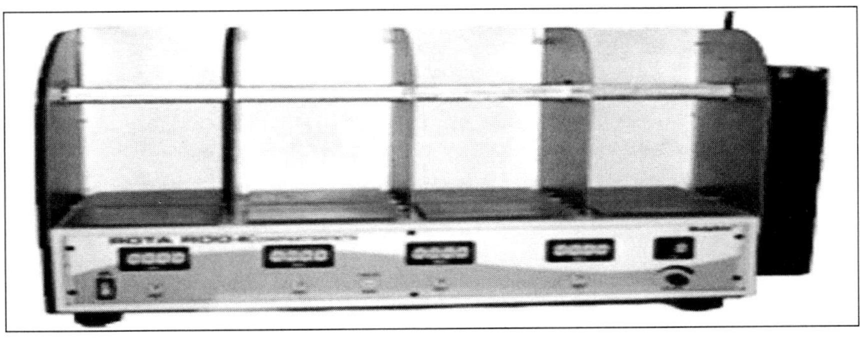

**Rotarod Apparatus**

## Specifications:

- Rotarod apparatus consists of a metal axle with a horizontal iron rod.
- The rod is divided into 2-5 sections for studying the muscle gripping activity in more number of animals (Mouse/Rat) at a time.
- Timer is placed in each section at the base of the instrument.
- The rod rotates at variable speed (20-25 rpm is ideal one).
- The retention time (sec) for each animal is recorded.
- The animal is trained to remain on the rod for 5 minutes and then the animal is administered a drug or vehicle and after 30 minutes again placed on apparatus and note the time.

## Applications:

- Rotarod apparatus is used to study muscle relaxant activity or the muscle grip of strength of drug in mice or rats.
- This instrument is used to study the effect of drug on motor co-ordination.
- An animal will fall immediately if the drug produces motor un-coordination, i.e. neurological deficit.
- It is used to measure balance, physical condition and motor planning.

## 3. Actophotometer:

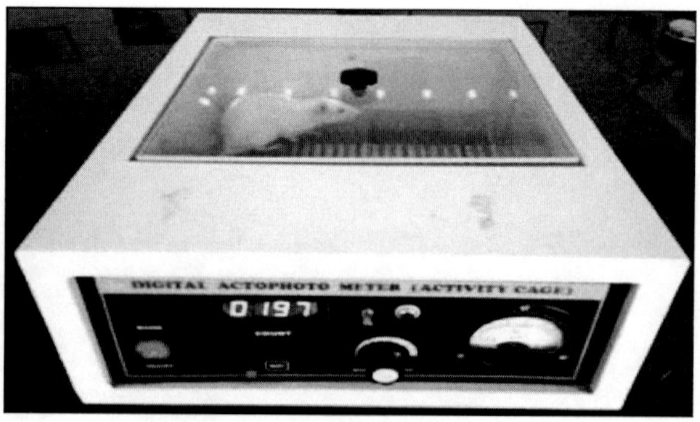


**Actophotometer**

## Specifications:

- Actophotometer consist of 30 cm long and 30 cm deep box with iron at the bottom.
- It operates on photoelectric cells in which six numbers of light and six numbers of photo cells are connected in circuit with an automatic counter.

- A photo cell is activated when the rays of light falling on the photo cells are cut-off by animal while crossing the beam of light and counter counts the number of cut-offs.
- One mouse can block only one beam of light at a time.

### Applications:

- Actophotometer or the activity cage or activity monitor is used to study the CNS stimulant and CNS depressant effect of the drug in mice and rats.
- This instrument is used to measure the motor activity of animals.
- It can measure both horizontal and perpendicular movements.
- The interruption of light beam activates a counter.
- The activity cage is used in toxicological, behavioural and psychopharmacological studies.

## 4. Elevated plus-maze:

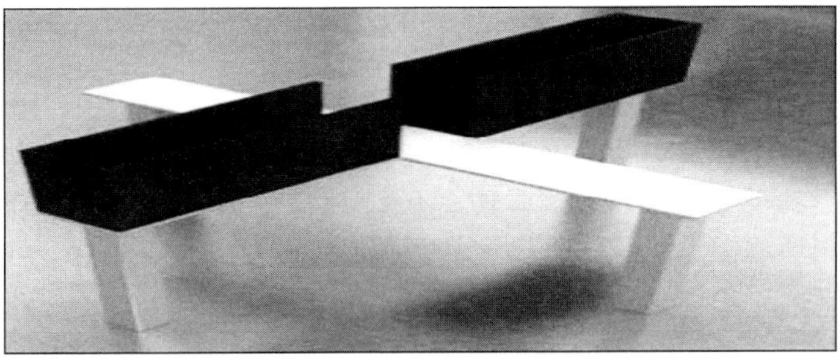

**Elevated plus-maze**

### Specifications:

- The plus-maze apparatus consists of two arms (16x5 cm for mouse and 50x10 cm for rats; LxW).
- Two enclosed arms (16x5x12 cm for mouse and 50x10x40 cm for rats; LxWxH), open to the top, and arranged such that the two open arms are opposite to each other.
- The maze is elevated to a height of 25 cm for mice and 50 cm for rats from the floor.

### Applications:

- Elevated plus-maze apparatus is used for screening of anxiolytic agents in mice and rats.
- It is most popularly used because of more simple apparatus, reliable, less time consuming.

- Rats and mice have dislike for high and open space and therefore they prefer enclosed arm so abnormality will observed.
- When animals enter open arm, they become immobile, freeze, defecate, have fear like movements and also plasma cortisol level is reported to increase which means the animal is having anxiety.
- Screening of motor activity and open arm exploratory time is also registered.
- Benzodiazepines and other anxiolytic decrease motor activity and increase open arm exploratory time.

## 5. Eddy's hot plate:

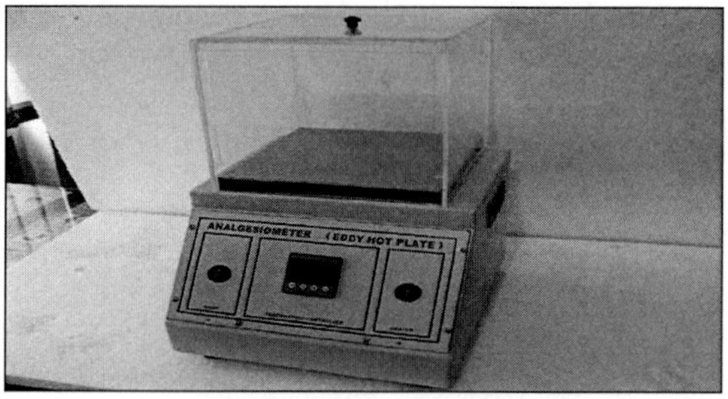


**Eddy's hot plate**

### Specifications:

- The eddy's hot plate is a surface of metal (10x10 cm) heated electrically to maintain a temperature of about 55 °C and covered from all the sides by perplex material.
- The animal is gently placed on the hot plate and time required to lick and jump response is noted down.
- The cut-off time is 20 seconds to avoid damage to the nerve ending of the paw, i.e., the experiment is terminated at 20 second and analgesia is considered as 100 percent.
- The paws of mice and rats are very sensitive to heat at temperature which are not damaging the skin.
- The hot plate method deals on the principle of thermal radiation.

### Applications:

- Hot plate is used for screening the central analgesic activity of drug in rats and mice.
- The conventional hot plate is used to carry out rapid screening of analgesic like morphine, codeine.
- It is also used in screening of anaesthetic response.

## 6. Electro- convulsiometer

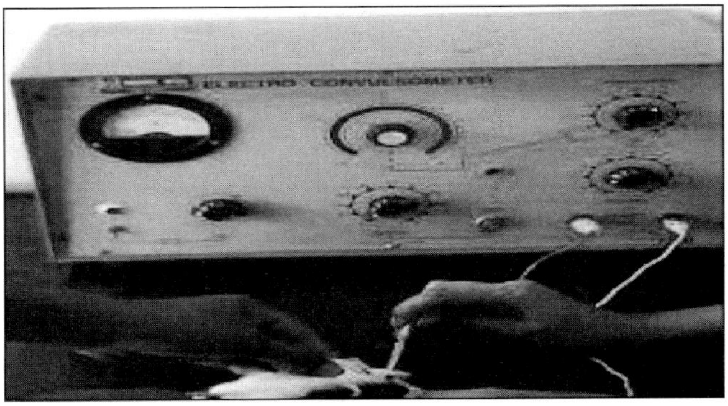

**Electro- convulsiometer**

### Specifications:

- Electro-convulsiometer is supplied with corneal electrodes of three different sizes specially developed for the application.
- Further, instrument is also supplied with ear electrode with tension adjusted to such a level to not cause any damage to rodent ear and also has insulation arrangement to protect the user.
- The instrument provides 50Hz stimulus current which can be adjusted from 0.15mA to 330mA in discrete steps for producing minimal and supra maximal seizures required in the assaying of anti-epileptic and anti-convulsant drugs.
- The application of stimulus current can be controlled by an electronic timer from 0.1second to 1 second in steps of 0.1 to 3 seconds in 11 steps. An L.E.D. indicates the duration of stimulus

### Applications:

- Electro-convulsiometer is used for applying maximal electro-shock through corneal electrodes provided.
- Instrument is used to study the anti-convulsant activity of phenytoin against maximal electro-shock induced convulsions in rat or mice. The instrument is provided with ammeter to control current intensity, timer & corneal electrodes.

## 7. Analgesiometer (Tail-flick method):

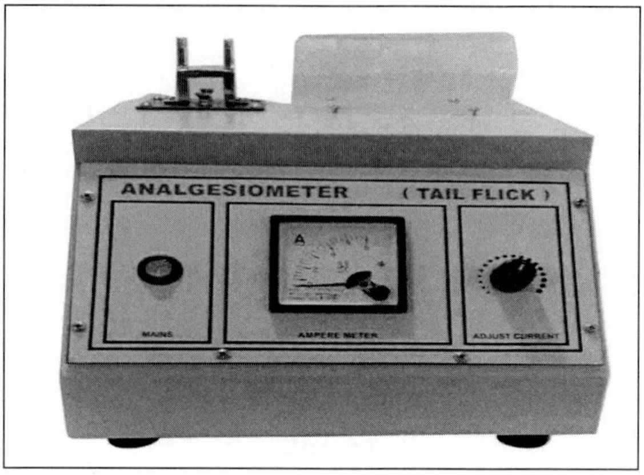


**Analgesiometer (Tail-flick method)**

### Specifications:

- Should consist of an I.R. source, whose radiant energy of adjustable intensity is focused on the rat tail.
- Restrainers should be available to be used with rat and mice.
- The digital instrument should automatically detect the withdrawal latency to the nearest 0.1 s.
- It provides pain stimulus by heated nichrome wire in a Rat's tail to determine analgesic effect of drugs. Complete with one spare element to work on 220 A.C.
- A radiant heat automatic tail flick analgesiometer was applied to measure reaction latencies.
- Basal reaction time of animals to radiant was recorded by locating the tip (last 1-2 cm) of the tail on radiant heat source.

### Applications:

- The tail flick method was utilized to study the antinociceptive activity in mice.
- Analgesiometer is used for screening the analgesic activity of drug in rats and mice.
- Analgesiometer is used to carry out rapid screening of analgesics like morphine, codeine.
- It is also used in screening of anaesthetic response.

# VIVA-VOCE

**Q.1 Write down the types of levers.**

**Ans: Types of lever:**

**I. Isotonic type:**

Change in length due to contraction is recorded while the tension on the muscle remains the same. Examples of isotonic levers are simple lever, frontal writing lever.

**II. Isometric type:**

Isometric recording measures increases in tension of the tissue when the length of the tissue is kept constant.

**The common recording levers used in the laboratory are:**

A. **Simple lever (side-way writing):** It is the simplest type of lever made up of wood, stainless steel or aluminium. A celluloid writing tip (stylus) is attached at the end of the longer arm. The contractions are recorded as curved lines.
B. **Frontal writing lever (writes frontally):** This lever is designed in such a way that the writing point rotates freely about its axle. This helps in reducing the tension between the smoked paper and the recording tip. The contractions are recorded as straight line.
C. **Starling's heart lever:** This lever is used to record the contraction of the heart. The difference between this and other isotonic levers is that the fulcrum lies at one end beyond the point of attachment.
D. **Brodie's universal lever:** It is a general utility lever having axis screwed with two nuts between which the interchangeable levers are clamped.

**Q.2 Write down the parts of lever.**

**Ans: Parts of lever**:

a. Effort arm: Point where force is to be applied
b. Load arm: Effect observed due to application of force.

**Q.3 Give different types of instruments used in experimental pharmacology.**

**Ans: Different types of instruments used in experimental pharmacology:**

- Sherrington recording drum and student's organ bath
- Eddy's hot plate
- Elevated plus maze
- Actophotometer
- Rota-rod Appratus
- Analgesiometer (Tail-flick method)
- Electro- convulsiometer

# Experiment No. 3

## Object: To study common laboratory animals.

## Introduction:

The use of animals in research and education dates back to the period when humans started to look for ways to prevent and cure ailments. Most of present day's drug discoveries were possible because of the use of animals in research.

Animal experimentation is the term used to explain the use of animals in experimentation in education, training and research. The terms animal testing, animal experimentation, animal research, in vivo testing and vivisection are often used interchangeably although they carry different meanings. "Vivisection", a term preferred by those who oppose the use of animals in research, means cutting into or dissecting a living animal. Researchers prefer to use the term 'animal experimentation'.

About 50-100 million animals ranging from zebra fish to non-human primates are used for experimentation every year. While experiments of vertebrates are regulated in most countries, those on invertebrates are not, and hence their accurate usage statistics are lacking.

The number of animals used in teaching varies from 1% to 10% of total animals used. Most of the animals used are small rodents. These are mostly used for fundamental biological research and breeding purposes. Most animals are used in only one procedure and are less commonly reused. These laboratory animals are obtained from various sources in different countries. The sources also vary based on species required. These experimental animals are mostly obtained through breeders. However, at some places these animals might be caught from the wild areas or from auctions. In India, animals have been mostly provided by small time traders, until a few years ago, after the CPCSEA guidelines were modified and affected, which bans the procurement of animals from unauthorized sources.

- Animal experimentation has been a part of biomedical and behavioral research for several millennia; experiments with animals were conducted in Greece over 2,000 years ago. Laboratory animals are used for different studies. It includes bioassay, preclinical studies.
- The use of an animal phylogenetically similar to man.

## Classifications:

**Rodents:** Ex. Mouse, Rats, Guinea Pig, Hamster.

**Non-Rodents:** Ex. Rabbits, Dog, Cat, Monkey, Pigs.

**Miscellaneous:** Ex. Frog, Pigeon, Zebra fish.

**Descriptions:** The commonly used laboratory animals in pharmacology laboratory are frog, rat, mice, guinea pig, hamster and rabbit. Cats and dogs are used to study the blood pressure experimental protocol. Monkey, pigs and some other animals were also used earlier, but now their use has been banned.

### 1. Mouse:

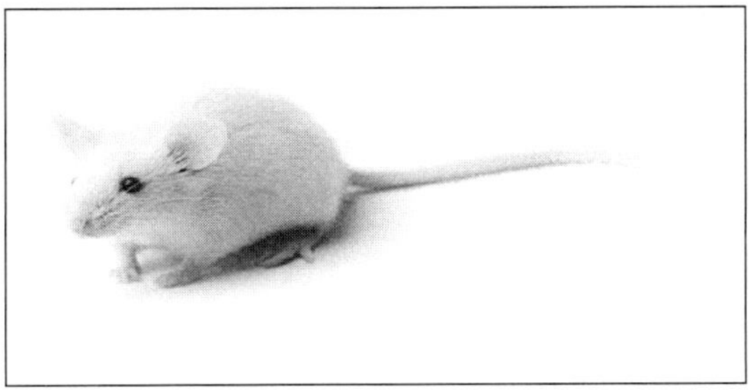

**Mice**

Mice are warm blooded rodent which are smallest laboratory animal. Mice are easy to breed and maintain. In biomedical research mice are preferred over other species because they are cheap and easy to handle. They require small space for housing and very sensitive to very small doses of drug substances.

### Applications:

- Rodents are small, easily housed and maintained, and adapt well to new surroundings.
- They also reproduce quickly and have a short lifespan of two to three years, so several generations of mice can be observed in a relatively short period of time.
- Used in toxicity study, bioassay(insulin), testing analgesics, CNS active drugs
- Immuno-deficient mice are boon for cancer and AIDS research.
- Around 2700 transgenic(Knock-in and knock-out) are available
- Low cost of maintenance and its ability to quickly multiply, reproducing as often as every nine weeks.
- Commonly used is swiss albino mice.

### Experimental Uses:

1. Toxicological studies
2. Teratogenicity studies
3. Bioassay of insulin, screening of analgesic and anticonvulsant drugs
4. Screening of chemotherapeutic agents
5. Studies related to genetics and cancer research

### Experimental procedures:

- Subcutaneous inoculation and Intra-peritoneal inoculation
- Intracerebral inoculation and Intravenous inoculation
- Intranasal inoculation and Collection of blood

## 2. Rat:

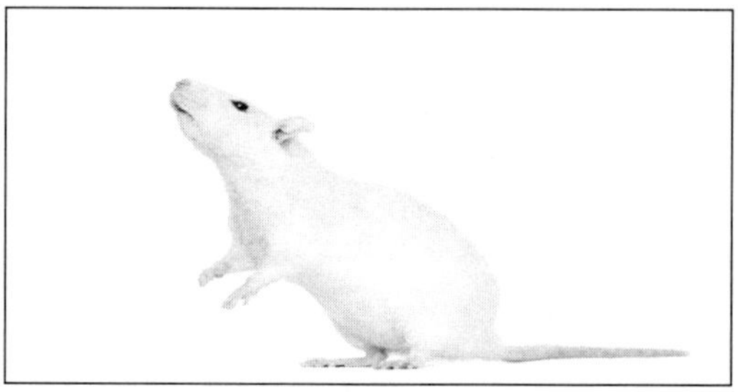

**Rat**

Rat is a warm blooded rodent which is the most common used animal for biomedical research. Rat does not vomit due to strong sphincter between stomach and esophagus and lack of vomiting center and tight presence of lower esophageal sphincter. It has no tonsils and gall bladder. It has diffuse pancreas, thus difficult to perform pancreactomy to induce type 1 diabetes mellitus. Rat is a coprophagousy animal who eat their own stool. Oestrus cycle appears at puberty at the age of two to three months and cycle lasts for about four to five days. The tail of rats is used for thermoregulation.

### The cycle is divided into four stages:

Estrus: It lasts for 9-15 h, It ends with ovulation.

Met-estrus: It is about 20 h and occurs shortly after ovulation.

Di-estrus: It is longest phase of about 60-70 h.

Pro-estrus: It last for about 12 h.

### Commonly used type:

**Wistar rats:** They have wide head; tail length is less than whole body length.

**Sprague dawley:** Narrow and long head, the tail length is greater than whole body length.

### Applications:

- Study of analgesics and anticonvulsants
- Study of oestrus cycle, mating behaviour and lactation
- Gastric acid secretion
- Hepatotoxicity studies.
- Bioassay of various hormones, such as insulin, oxytocin, vasopressin
- Toxicology studies
- Rat brain tissue is extensively employed in radio-receptor ligand studies.

## 3. Guinea Pig:

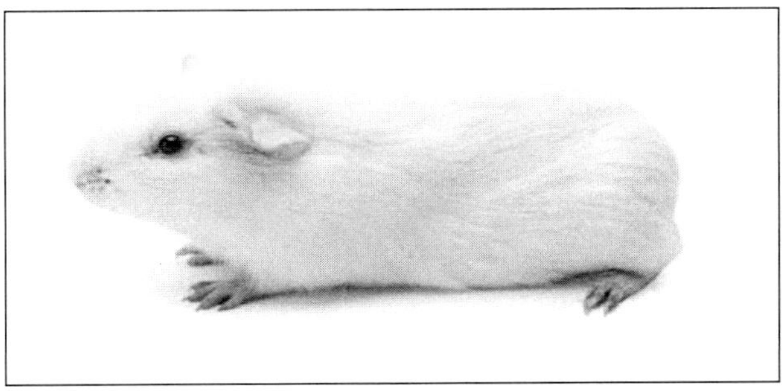

**Guinea Pig**

Guinea pig is a warm blooded rodent, very docile and easy to raise and maintain laboratory animals. It is herbivorous animal and daily requires vitamin C in diet like human. Guinea pig is highly sensitive to histamine. They are therefore, used in experimental asthma to study bronchodilators. They are very susceptible to tuberculosis and anaphylactic shock. They are also used to study local anaesthetics and as model in experimental amoebiasis and cholera as they are sensitive to these microorganisms. Penicillin is more toxic to guinea pig than to the mouse. Guinea pig isolated heart and '-achea are sensitive to histamine. Guinea pig serum contains an enzyme asparaginase, which has antileukemic action.

### Applications:

- Vaccines for diphtheria and tuberculosis
- Hypersensitivity studies

- Anaphylactic shock
- Evaluation of bronchodilators
- Evaluation of local anaesthetics
- Terminal portion of ileum used for screening spasmodic and anti spasmodic agents
- Nutritional studies (Ascorbic acid metabolism)

### Experimental procedures:

- Anasthesia (Pentobarbitone sodium 28mg/kg-body weight).
- Subcutaneous inoculation.
- Intracutaneous inoculation.
- Intraperitoneal inoculation.
- Collection of blood.

## 4. Rabbit:

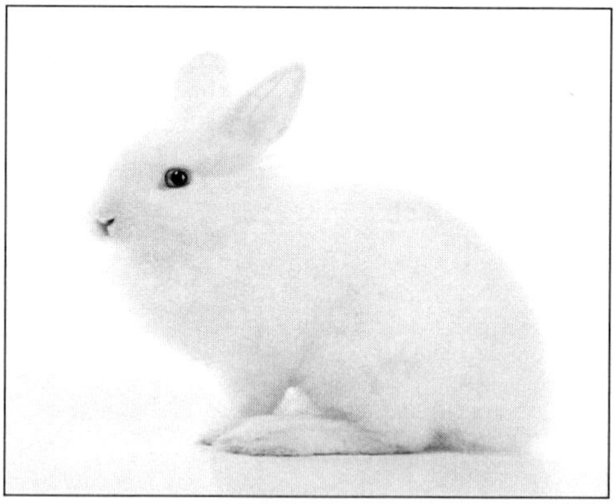

**Rabbit**

Rabbit is warm blooded mammalian and a docile animal used for various studies. Domestic rabbits are generally used for pyrogen testing. Some strains of rabbit are resistant to the effect of atropine because they have high concentration of atropinesterase enzymes in their blood. Some of the tissue or organs from rabbits used are heart, aorta, duodenum and ileum. In rabbits coitus itself induces secretion of leutenising hormones in females, which leads to the ovulation. Progesterone is known to block ovulation.

### Applications:

- Rabbits are commonly used for toxicity and safety testing of substances such as drugs, chemicals and medical devices.

- They are used in skin and eye irritation studies, such as the archaic and painful Draize tests for cosmetics, personal care, household products and other chemicals.
- A number of rabbit models have been developed to study human diseases, the most common being cardiovascular disease, cancer and AIDS. They have also been used as bioreactors for the production of pharmaceutical proteins.
- Testing of large volume parentrals, screening and bioassay of insulin
- Antihyperglycemics
- Pyrogen testing
- Testing Topical agents as skin is sensitive
- Bioassay of anti-diabetic drugs, insulin, curare mimetic drugs
- Studies related to anti-fertility agents
- It has simple cardiac tissue free of connective tissue and hence is the animal of choice for cardiac studies
- Screening embryotoxic agents and teratogens

**Experimental procedures:**

- Subcutaneous inoculation
- Intra-venous inoculation
- Intra-peritoneal inoculation
- Intra-cerebral inoculation
- Ophthalmic
- Collection of blood

## 5. Frog:

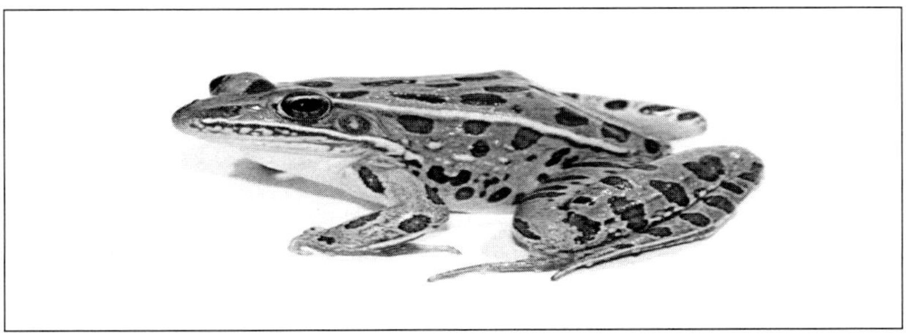

**Frog**

Frogs (150-200g) were one time extensively used in experimental pharmacology. However, recently the use of wild frogs for experimental purposes has been banned. Earlier, frogs were used for isolated heart, rectus abdominis muscle preparation, study of muscle nerve and ciliary movements, respectively. Frogs were also used for the study of nerve block type of local anaesthetics. Frogs are inexpensive and easily available, and the ban on the use of frogs has been debated.

## 6. Hamster:

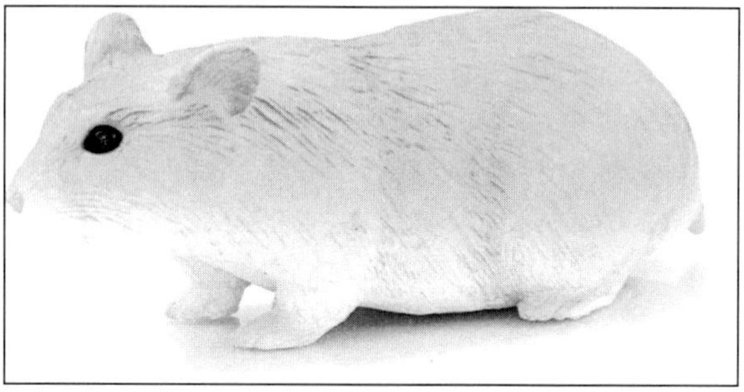

**Hamster**

Hamster have short body with short legs and tail. The skin is loose and covered with dense short soft fur. The cheek pouches are prominent and extend up to the shoulder region.

### Applications:

- Chines hamsters have low chromosome number making it useful for cytological investigations, genetics, tissue culture and radiation research.
- Research on diabetes mellitus.
- Research related to virology, immunology and implantation studies.
- Bioassay of prostaglandins.

## Other animals:

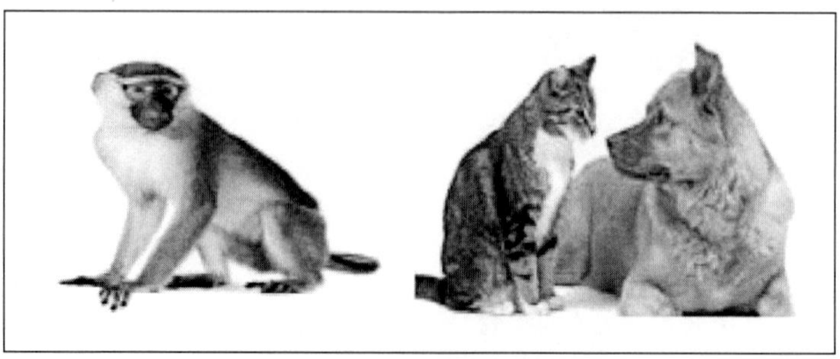

**Monkey, Cat and Dog**

Cats, dogs and monkeys are used for pharmacological investigations of drugs. Cats and dogs were one time commonly used to study blood pressure experiments. But their use has now been restricted. However beagle dogs are the only strain approved by regulatory authorities (USFDA) for preclinical testing of new drugs. Chronically prepared fistula and pouches of dogs are used to study the gastric secretory function. Monkeys are not used for routine pharmacological testing. Since they constitute one of the subhuman mammals closest to man in many aspects, the toxicity study on monkeys forms an essential requirement for developing a new drug for human use. Monkeys are quite expensive and difficult to breed and maintain.

**Table: Some Physiological Data on Laboratory Animals**

| S.No. | Parameters | Rat | Mouse | Rabbit | Guinea pig | Dog |
|---|---|---|---|---|---|---|
| 1. | Body weight (gm) | 200-300 | 25-30 | 2000-3000 | 500-800 | 5000-8000 |
| 2. | Life span (yrs) | 2-3 | 1-2 | 4-5 | 2 | Up to 10 |
| 3. | Water consumption (ml/d) | 35 | 6 | 200-300 | 250-350 | 500-700 |
| 4. | Food consumption (g/d) | 20 | 5 | 100 | 30 | 500 |
| 5. | Urine excretion (ml/d) | 10-15 | 1-3 | 200-300 | 100-150 | 600-700 |
| 6. | Oestrus cycle (d) | 4-5 | 4-5 | Spontaneous ovulator | 15-19 | 180 |
| 7. | Gestation period (d) | 21 | 19 | 32 | 67 | 62 |
| 8. | Breeding age (d) | 60-80 | 42-56 | 90-120 | 365 | 90 |
| 9. | Breeding life (yrs) | 1-1.25 | 0.75-1.5 | 3 | 1 | 6-7 |
| 10. | Litter size | 10-12 | 10-12 | 4-8 | 2-4 | 2-6 |
| 11. | Body temperature (°C) | 37.5 | 37.4 | 38.3 | 38.3 | 37.7 |
| 12. | Respiratory rate (Breaths/min) | 80-150 | 90-180 | 35-60 | 60-110 | 14-28 |
| 13. | Heart-rate (Beats/min) | 260-450 | 300-750 | 205-308 | 250-300 | 77-138 |
| 14. | Blood pressure (mmHg) | 130/90 | 120/75 | – | – | 140/80 |
| 15. | Blood volume (ml/kg) | 50-65 | 70-80 | 45-70 | 65-90 | 75-100 |
| 16. | Room temperature (°C) | 24-27 | 24-27 | 24-27 | 24-27 | 24-27 |
| 17. | Relative humidity % | 50-60 | 50-60 | 70 | 60-70 | 60-70 |

## VIVA-VOCE

**Q.1 Give the classification of experimental animals.**

**Ans:** Classifications:

Rodents: Ex. Mouse, Rats, Guinea Pig, Hamster.

Non-Rodents: Ex. Rabbits, Dog, Cat, Monkey, Pigs.

Miscellaneous: Ex. Frog, Pigeon, Zebra fish.

**Q.2 Give the experimental uses of laboratory animals.**

**Ans:** The use of animals in experimentation in education, training and research. The terms animal testing, animal experimentation, animal research, in vivo testing and vivisection are often used interchangeably although they carry different meanings.

# Experiment No. 4

## Object: To study the maintenance of laboratory animals as per CPCSEA guidelines.

### Introduction:

#### The Committee for the Purpose of Control and Supervision of Experiments on Animals (CPCSEA):

The Committee for the Purpose of Control and Supervision of Experiments on Animals (CPCSEA) is a statutory Committee, which is established under Chapter 4, Section 15(1) of the Prevention of Cruelty to Animals Act 1960.

India is one of the pioneering countries to institute Prevention of Cruelty to Animals Act in 1960 whereas such Act was instituted in France in 1963 and in USA in 1966. The detailed rules for experimentation on animals were first enacted by the Ministry of Agriculture in 1968 and were implemented by a Committee set up in pursuance of Section 15(1) of the PCA Act, 1960.

However, the Committee was later wound up in 1977. After a hiatus of 13 years, a recommendation to reconstitute Committee for the purpose of control and supervision of experiments on animals (CPCSEA) was received from Animal Welfare Board of India (AWBI). After due consideration of the recommendation of AWBI, CPCSEA was set up by this Ministry on 8th February, 1991.

The Committee was, subsequently, reconstituted on 23rd February, 1996 with 15 Members and one Member Secretary. Since then, this Ministry has reconstituted the CPCSEA routinely. The present Committee was constituted on 30th August, 2012 under the chairmanship of Additional Secretary, MoEF with 17 Members. At present, Shri Hem Pande, Additional Secretary, MoEF & CC is the Chairman of the Committee.

#### The functions of CPCSEA:

1. Registration of establishments conducting animal experimentation or breeding of animals for this purpose.
2. Selection and assignment of nominees for the Institutional Animal Ethics Committees of the registered establishments.
3. Approval of Animal House Facilities on the basis of reports of inspections conducted by CPCSEA.
4. Permission for conducting experiments involving use of animals.
5. Recommendation for import of animals for use in experiments.

6. Action against establishments. In case of established, violation of any legal norm/ stipulation.
7. Conduct of Training Programmes for the Nominees of CPCSEA.
8. Conduct / Support of Conference / workshop on Animal Ethics.

## Maintenance of laboratory animals as per CPCSEA guideline:

- The goal of these guidelines is to promote the human care of animal used in biomedical and behavioural research and testing.
- To avoid unnecessary pain before, during and after experiment.
- To provide guideline for:
  - Housing, care, breeding and maintenance
  - Source of experimental animals
  - Acceptable experimental procedures for anesthesia and euthanasia

  It is essential to take care of below mentioned points regarding the experimentation on animal as per CPCSEA guideline:

## Animal Procurement:

1. Quarantine
2. Stabilization
3. Separation

### 1. Quarantine:

- Separation of newly received animals from those already in the facility until the health and possibly the microbial status of newly received animal have been determined.
- A minimum duration of quarantine for small animal-1 week and for larger animal-6 week.

### 2. Stabilization:

- Physiologic, psychological and nutritional stabilization should be given before their use.
- Duration of stabilization will depend on type and duration of animal transportation, and species of animal.

### 3. Separation:

- Physical separation of animal by species is recommended to prevent interspecies disease transmission and to eliminate anxiety and possible physiological and behavioural changes due to interspecies conflict.

- Housing different species in separate room.
- It shall be acceptable to house different species in the same room, e.g. two species have a similar pathogen status and are behaviourally compatible.

## Surveillance, Diagnosis, Treatment and Control of Disease:

- All animals should be observed for signs of illness, injury, or abnormal behaviour by animal house staff.
- Animals that show signs of a contagious disease should be isolated from healthy animals in the colony.

## Animal care and technical personnel:

- Animal care require technical and husbandry support.
- Institution should employ people trained in laboratory animal or provide for both formal and on the job training to ensure effective implementation of the program.

## Personal Hygiene:

- Animal care staff maintain a high standard of personal cleanliness.
- Clothing suitable for use in the animal facility should be supplied and laundered by the institution.
- It is acceptable to use disposable gear such as gloves, masks, head covers, coats, coveralls and shoe covers.
- Person should change clothing as often as is necessary to maintain personal hygiene.
- Personnel should not be permitted to eat, drink, smoke or apply cosmetic in animal rooms.

## Multiple surgical procedures on single animal:

- Multiple surgical procedures on a single animal for any testing or experiment are not to be practiced unless specified in a protocol only approved by the IAEC.

## Duration of experiments:

- No animal should be used for experimentation for more than 3 years unless adequate justification is provided.

## Physical restraint:

- Restraint devices cannot be used simply as a convenience in handling or managing animals.

- The period of restraint should be the minimum required to accomplish the research objectives.
- Provision should be made for observation of the animal at appropriate intervals.

## Physical relationship of animal facilities of laboratories:

- Animal shall be housed in an isolated building located as far away from human habitations as possible and not exposed to dust, smoke, noise, wild rodent, insects and birds.
- This separation can be accomplished by having the animal quarters in a separate building, wing, floor or room.
- The animal room should occupy about 50-60% of the total constructed area and the remaining area should be utilized for service such as stores, washing, office and staff, machine rooms, quarantine and corridors.
- Since animals are very sensitive to environmental changes, sharp fluctuations in temperature, humidity, light, sound and ventilation should be avoided.

## Functional areas:

- Ensure separation of species or isolation of individual projects when necessary.
- Receiving and storage areas for food, bedding.
- Space for administration, supervision, and direction of the facility.
- Showers, sinks, lockers and toilets for personnel.
- Washing and sterilization equipment and supplies.
- For holding soiled and cleaned equipment.
- For repairing cages and equipment.
- To store wastes prior to incineration or removal.

## Physical facilities:

### 1. Building Materials:

Moisture-proof, fire-resistant, seamless materials are most desirable for interior surfaces including vermin and pest resistance.

### 2. Corridor:

Wide enough to facilitate the movement of personnel as well as equipments and should be kept clean.

### 3. Utilities:

Water lines, drain pipes and electrical connection.

### 4. Animal Room Doors:

Rust, vermin and dust proof, properly within their frames and provided with an observation window.

### 5. Floors:

Smooth, moisture proof, non-absorbent, skid-proof, resistant to wear, acid, solvents, adverse effects of detergents and disinfectants. Capable of supporting racks, equipment and stored items without becoming gouged, cracked, or pitted.

### 6. Drains:

Floor drains are not essential in all rooms used exclusively for housing rodents.

### 7. Walls & Ceilings:

Free of cracks, unsealed utility penetrations, or imperfect junction with doors, ceilings, floors and corners.

### 8. Storage Areas:

Separate storage areas should be designed for feed, bedding, cages and materials not in use.

### 9. Facilities for Sanitizing Equipment and Supplies:

An area for sanitizing cages and ancillary equipment is essential with adequate water supply.

### 10. Experimental Area:

It should be carried out in a separate area away from the place where animals are housed.

## Environment:

### 1. Temperature and Humidity control:

- Air conditioning
- Temperature with in the range of 64.4-84.0 F
- Relative humidity- 30-70% throughout the year
- For large animal comfortable zone-18-37°c

### 2. Power and Lighting:

- The electrical system should be safe and provide appropriate lighting and a sufficient no. of power outlets.
- A time control light system should be used.

### 3. Noise Control:

- Noise free environment

## Animal Husbandry Caging & Housing System:

- Adequate ventilation
- Meet the biological need of animal
- Keep the animal dry and clean
- Facilitate research while maintaining good health of the animals
- Cages made of steel or painted steel
- Feeding and watering devices should be easily accessible for filing, changing, cleaning and servicing.

## Food:

- It should be fed palatable, non-contaminated and nutritionally adequate food.
- Feeders should allow easy access to food while avoiding contamination by urine and faeces.
- Food should be available in a mount sufficient to ensure normal growth in immature animals and maintenance of normal body weight, reproduction and lactation in adults.
- Areas in which diets are stored should be kept clean and enclosed to prevent entry of insects or other animals.
- Diet should be free from heavy metals.

## Bedding:

- Absorbent, free of toxic chemicals or other substances that could injure animals or personnel, and of a type not readily eaten by animals.
- It should be removed and replaced with fresh materials as often as necessary to keep animal clean and dry.
- It should be easily stored.
- Uncontaminated
- Non-toxic
- Non-malodorous
- Disposable by incineration

## Water:

- Fresh
- Potable
- Uncontaminated

## Water Disposal:

- The most preferred method of waste disposal is incineration.
- If wastes must be stored before removal, the waste storage area should be separated from other storage facilities and free of flies, cockroaches, rodents and other vermin.

## Pest Control:

- Programs designed to prevent, control, or eliminate the presence of or infestations by pests are essential in an animal environment.

## Emergency, Weekend and Holiday care:

- Animal should be cared for by qualified personnel every day, including weekends and holidays, to safeguard their well- being including emergency veterinary care.

## Record Keeping:

- Animal house plans
- Animal house staff record
- Health record of staff/animals
- All SOPs relevant to the animals
- Breeding, stock, purchase and sales records
- Minutes of institute animal ethics committee meetings
- Record of experiments conducted with the no. of animals used
- Death record
- Clinical record of sick animals, training record of staff involved in animal activities.
- Water analysis report

## Standard Operating Procedures (SOPs)/ Guidelines:

- Maintain SOPs describing procedures/ methods adapted with regard to animal husbandry, maintenance, breeding, animal house microbial analysis and experimentation record.

- SOPs should contain following items-
  - Name of author
  - Title of SOP
  - Date of preparation
  - Reference of previous SOP on the same subject and date
  - Location and distribution of SOPs with sign of each recipient
  - Objectives
  - Detailed information of the instruments used in relation with animals
  - Normal value of all parameters.

## Transport of Laboratory Animals:

- The main considerations for transport of animals are the mode of transport, the containers, the animal density in cages, food and water during transit, protection from transit infection, injuries and stress.

## Anaesthesia:

- Sedatives, analgesics and anaesthetics should be used to control pain or distress under experiment. Before using actual anaesthetics the animals are prepared for anaesthesia by overnight fasting and using pre-anaesthetics.
- Local or general anaesthetics may be used depending on type of surgical procedure.

## Euthanasia:

- Sacrificing the experimental animals after their use by a gentle procedure causing minimum of physical and mental suffering is called euthanasia (painless killing).
- Physical methods of euthanasia include stunning, cervical dislocation, decapitation and microwave irradiation.
- The most suitable chemical euthanasia is through the use of certain anaesthetics in overdose.
- Injectable anaesthetics such as barbiturates (sodium pentobarbitone) are most widely used for euthanasia in experimental animals.
- Exposure of animals to carbon dioxide at high concentration (80-100%) causes unconsciousness followed by death within a few seconds and this method is also used for euthanasia.

## Disposal:

- The transgenic and knockout animal should be first euthanized and then disposed off as prescribed elsewhere in the guidelines.
- A record of disposal and the manner of disposal should be kept as a matter of routine.

# VIVA-VOCE

**Q.1 Write down the full form of CPCSEA.**

**Ans:** Committee for the Purpose of Control and Supervision of Experiments on Animals

**Q.2 Define Euthanasia.**

**Ans:** Sacrificing the experimental animals after their use by a gentle procedure causing minimum of physical and mental suffering is called euthanasia (painless killing).

**Q.3 Write down the functions of CPCSEA.**

**Ans: The functions of CPCSEA:**

1. Registration of establishments conducting animal experimentation or breeding of animals for this purpose.
2. Selection and assignment of nominees for the Institutional Animal Ethics Committees of the registered establishments.
3. Approval of Animal House Facilities on the basis of reports of inspections conducted by CPCSEA.
4. Permission for conducting experiments involving use of animals.
5. Recommendation for import of animals for use in experiments.
6. Action against establishments in case of established violation of any legal norm/ stipulation.
7. Conduct of Training Programmes for the Nominees of CPCSEA.
8. Conduct / Support of Conference / workshop on Animal Ethics.

# Experiment No. 5

## Object: To study the common laboratory techniques. Blood withdrawal, serum and plasma separation, anaesthetics and euthanasia used for animal studies.

### Introduction:

Blood collection from the experimental laboratory animals is one of the very important procedures of the biomedical research. For the wide range of research it is necessary to collect the blood from animals for different biochemical or haematological parameters and also measuring the concentration of drug in the blood for pharmacokinetics study. During collection of blood sample the very important thing is that the experimental animal should be in less stress because that stress will affect the study outcome. Permission from the Institute Animal Ethics Committee (IAEC) is required for blood withdrawal from laboratory animals.

### Principle:

- The collection process of blood sample should be less painful and stressful.
- If the experiments need multiple collection of blood then rabbit can be used.
- About 10% of total circulating blood volume can be withdrawn from healthy, normal, adult animal without causing considerable changes in its physiology and the animal should not bleed for 3 weeks at least in single withdrawn.
- If the blood collection exceeds 10% of total volume of blood then fluid replacement may be required.
- Special care should be taken for pregnant, obese and older animals.

| Species | Blood Volume Mean (ml/kg) | Blood Volume Range (ml/kg) | Blood Volume (average) | | |
|---|---|---|---|---|---|
| Mouse (25 g average Wt.) | 58.6 | 55-80 | 7.5% | 10% | 15% |
| Rat (250 g) | 64 | 58-70 | 1.2 ml | 1.6 ml | 2.4 ml |
| Rabbit (4 kg) | 56 | 44-70 | 17 ml | 22 ml | 34 ml |
| Nonhuman primate (NHP; 8 kg) | 56 | 55-75 | 34 ml | 45 ml | 67 ml |

| Single sampling | | Multiple sampling | |
|---|---|---|---|
| **% Circulatory blood volume removed** | **Approximate recovery period** | **% Circulatory blood volume removed (cumulative volume)** | **Approximate recovery Period** |
| 7.5% | 1 week | 7.5% | 1 week |
| 10% | 2 weeks | 10-15% | 2 weeks |
| 10-15% | 4 weeks | 20% | 3 weeks |

## Requirements:

**Animals:** Experimental laboratory animals.

**Drugs:** Anticoagulants, Anaesthesia.

**Equipments:** Restrainers, Syringe, Cotton, Surgical blade, Blood collection tube.

## Procedure:

1. **Non-terminal blood withdrawal:** In this the blood is collected from the conscious or unconscious experimental laboratory animals by single or multiple withdrawals. Animals are not sacrificed after blood collection.
2. **Terminal Blood withdrawal:** In this type, large volume of blood is withdrawn from animal from single or multiple withdrawals by giving anaesthesia to the experimental animals. After the blood is withdrawn the animals are sacrificed.

## Different techniques of blood withdrawal from laboratory animals:

### Non-terminal blood withdrawal procedure:

1. Tail vein
2. Orbital sinus
3. Marginal ear vein
4. Jugular vein
5. Tarsal vein
6. Blood vessel cannulation
7. Dorsal pedal

### Terminal Blood withdrawal procedure:

1. Cardiac Puncture
2. Posterior vena cava
3. Orbital sinus

## 1. Tail vein:

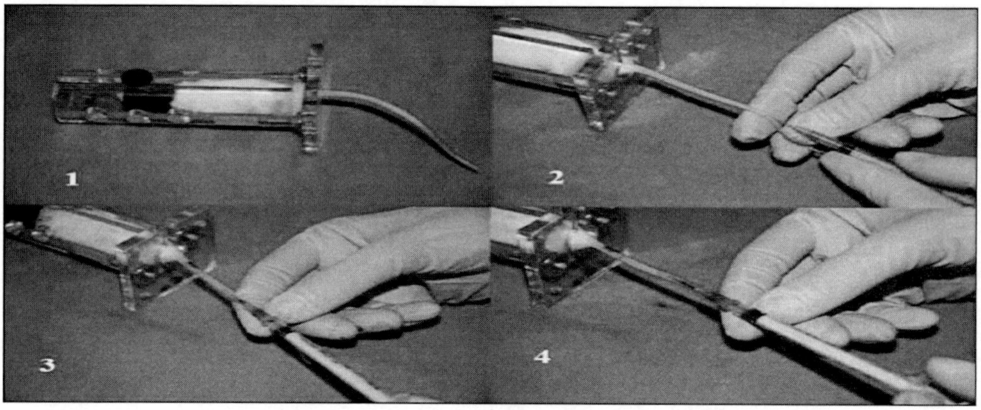


**Blood collection from the tail vein**

### Procedure:

- This process is carried on conscious rat/mice by applying the local anaesthesia cream on tail before 10 min of blood withdrawal.
- To increase blood circulation into the tail vein the tail is dipped in warm water. The needle (23-25 G) is inserted into the tail vein and blood is slowly withdrawn without interruption of vein.
- Another method for tail vein blood withdrawal is by cutting terminal part of the tail and giving the pressure on it.

### Advantage:

- This method is very easy to perform.
- This method gives lesser pain to the animals.

### Disadvantage:

- The amount of blood that can be withdrawn is very small.

## 2. Orbital Sinus or Retro-orbital Plexus Bleeding:

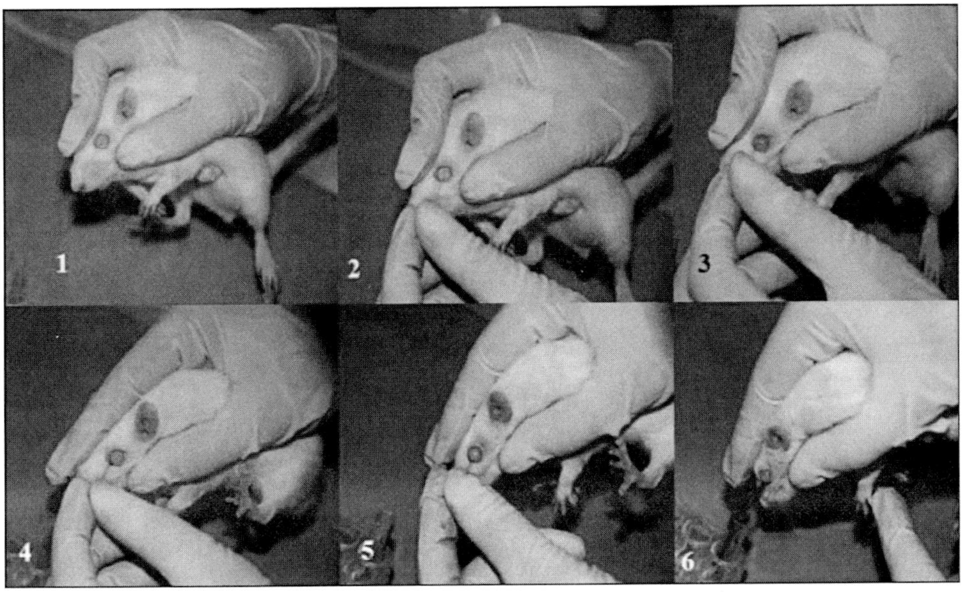


**Blood collection from the orbital sinus or retro-orbital plexus**

### Procedure:

- This procedure is carried out in rodents under ether anaesthesia.
- The animal is picked with thumb and index finger so the skin around the eye is stretched and clears the eye site.
- The fine capillary tube is inserted into medial canthus of the eye at 30 degree angle to the nose. Slight pressure is applied by rotating the capillary which is enough to puncture the tissue and enter into the plexus.
- The amount of blood required is collected and gently remove the capillary tube from the retro-orbital plexus. Bleeding can be stopped by applying cotton on eye sight of animal.

### Advantages:

- Larger amount of blood can be withdrawn.

### Disadvantages:

- This method requires skilful handling of the animal otherwise it may cause irreversible damage to the eyes of the animal

## 3. Marginal ear vein/Artery:

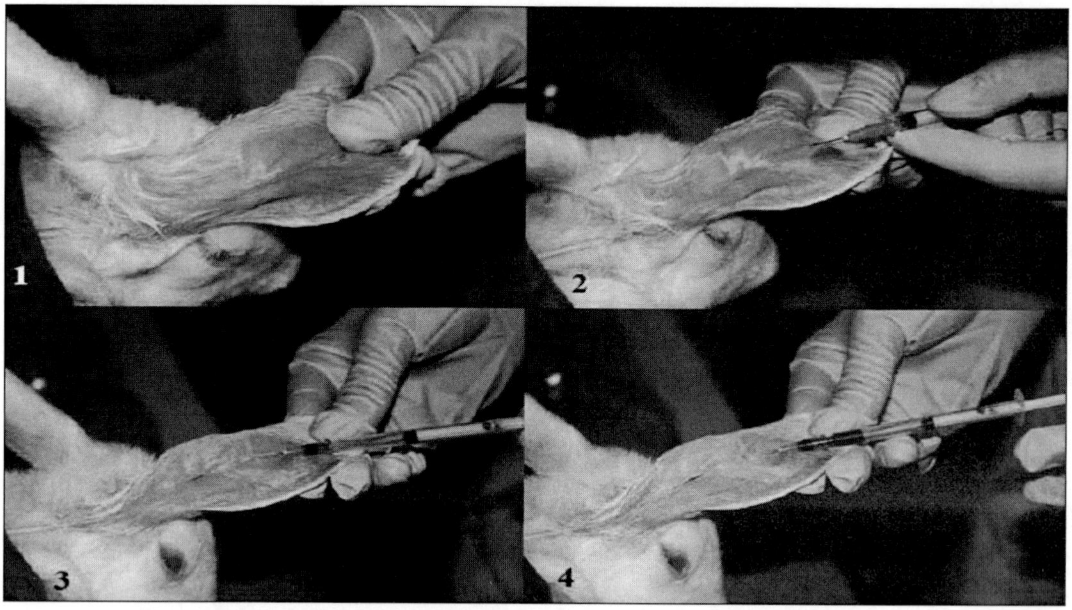

**Blood collection from the marginal ear vein/artery**

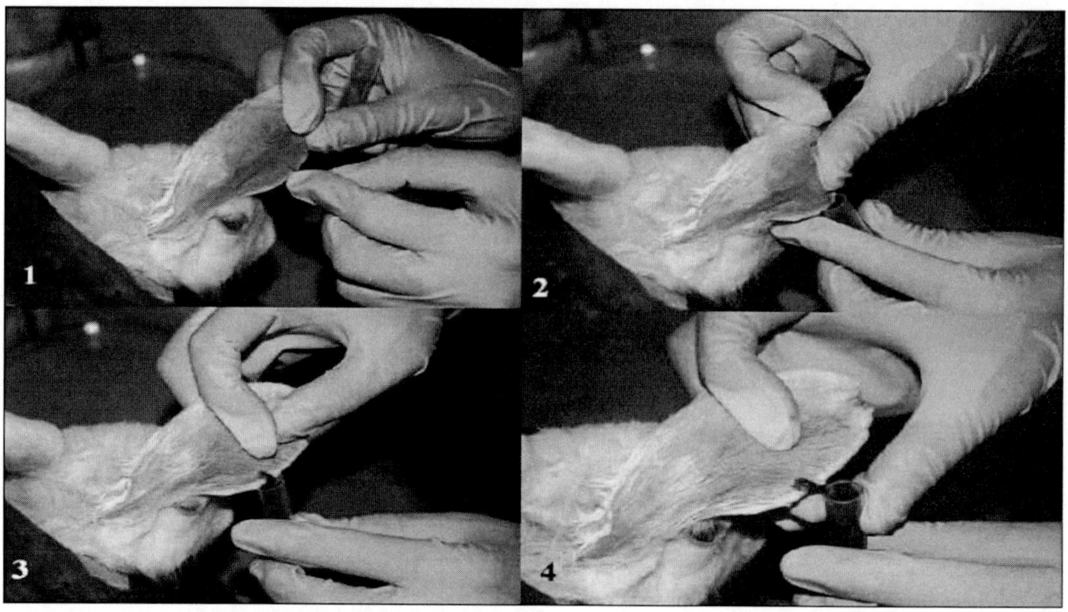

**Blood collection from the marginal ear vein/artery**

## Procedure:

- The rabbit should be placed properly in the holder by keeping head outside. Ear is cleaned gently with spirit or 90% alcohol and applying the local anaesthetic cream before 10 min of sampling.
- If dilation of blood vessel is required, topical vasodilator may be applied on collection sight. With the help of needle and syringe the blood is withdrawn. Bleeding can be stopped with the use of sterile cotton pressed on collection site.

## Advantages:

- Larger amount of blood can be withdrawn.
- Frequent blood withdrawal is possible.

## Disadvantages:

- Behavioural activity may be affect.
- These techniques want skilful person.

## 4. Jugular vein:

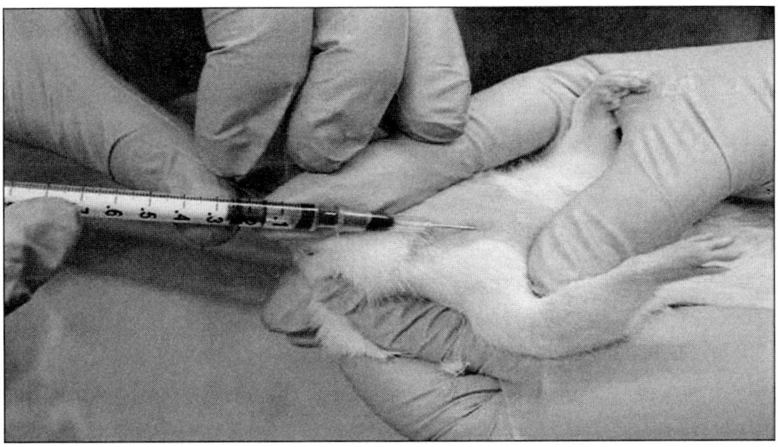

**Blood collection from the jugular vein**

## Procedure:

- In this method, warming of the animals is not required and is used to collect micro volumes to one ml of blood sample.
- This method has to be carried out under general/inhalation anesthesia and two persons are needed to collect blood sample.

- One person has to restrain the animal and monitor the animal. Another person is required to collect the blood sample from the animal.
- The neck region of the animal is shaved and kept in hyperextended position. The jugular veins appear blue in color and is found 2 to 4 mm lateral to sternoclavicular junction. A 25G needle is inserted in the caudocephalic direction (back to front) and blood is withdrawn slowly to avoid collapse of these small blood vessels. Animal has to be handled carefully and not more than 3 to 4 mm of needle is to be inserted into the blood vessel.
- If the attempt to collect blood fails, the needle is slowly removed and the site is monitored for bleeding. If there is no bleeding, one more attempt can be made. Further attempts should be avoided in case of bleeding as it may collapse the vein.
- Finger pressure is applied to stop bleeding.
- **Precaution:** Number of attempts is limited to three. Apply local anesthetic cream 30 minutes prior to sampling.

## 5. Tarsal vein:

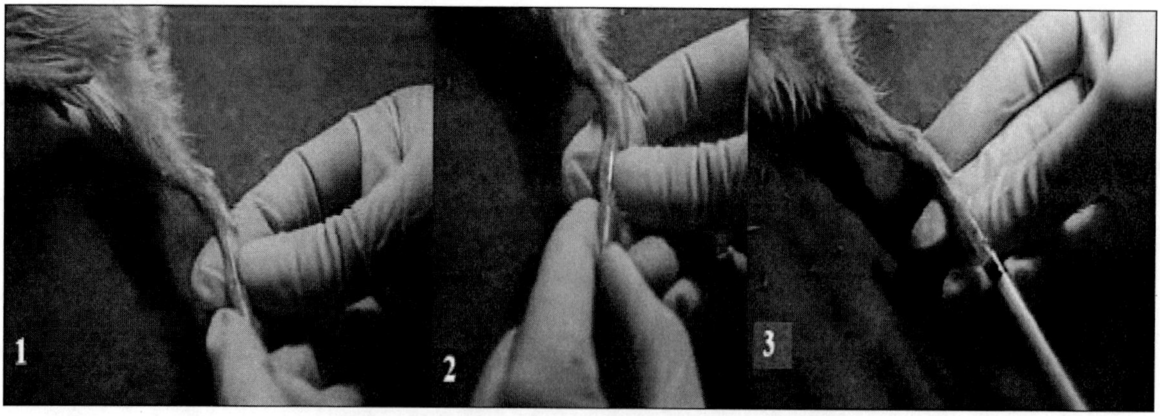


**Blood collection from the tarsal vein**

### Procedure:

- Tarsal vein is identified in one of the hind legs of large animals. This method is commonly recommended for guinea pig.
- One person has to restrain the animal properly. Tarsal vein may be visible in blue color. The surface hairs are removed by applying a suitable hair remover.
- A local anesthetic cream is applied on the collection site. After 20 to 30 minutes, blood sample is collected slowly by using 22G needle.

- Maximum three samples can be taken per leg and 0.1 to 0.3 ml of blood can be collected per sample. After the sample collection, gentle pressure is applied with finger for 2 minutes to stop bleeding
- **Precaution:** Not more than six samples from both hind legs are taken. The number of attempts is three or less.

## 6. Blood vessel cannulation:

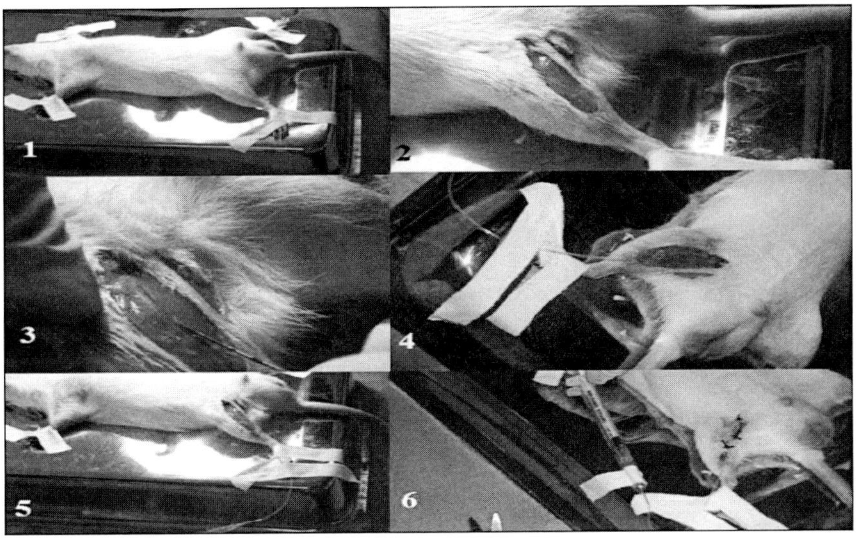


**Blood collection from the blood vessel cannulation**

### Procedure:

- This method involves continuous and multiple sampling in the experimental animal. This method requires close and continuous monitoring of the animal.
- Usually blood vessel cannulation is done in the femoral artery, femoral vein, carotid artery, jugular vein, vena cava and dorsal aorta. Surgery is required for this method and appropriate anesthesia and analgesia should be used to minimize the pain.
- After surgical cannulation, animal should be housed singly in a large and spacious cage. Blood sample may be collected over 24 hour at the volume of 0.1 to 0.2 ml/sample. After withdrawing the blood, the cannula is flushed with an anticoagulant and the withdrawn volume may be replaced (if required) with LRS and cannula should be closed tightly

- **Precaution:** The experiment has to be conducted fully under aseptic precautions. Infection, hemorrhage, blockage of cannula and swelling around the cannulation site should be looked for.

## 7. Dorsal Pedal:

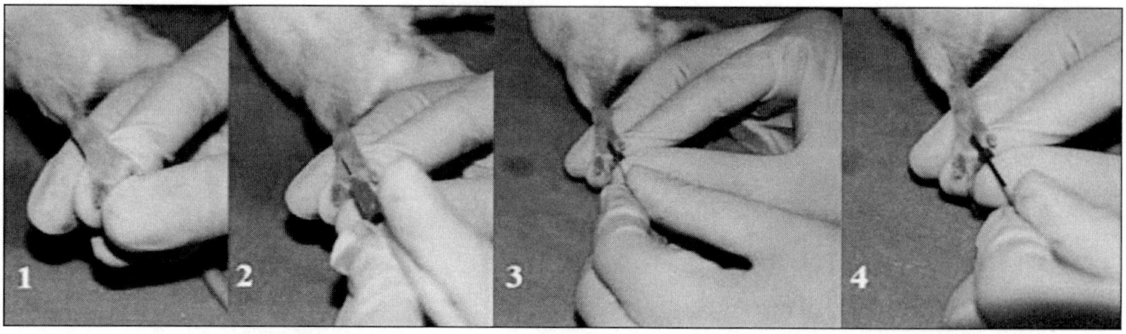


**Blood collection from the dorsal pedal**

### Procedure:

- This method is mainly carried out in rat or mice.
- The animal is kept in restrainer. The hind foot ankle is held and medial dorsal pedal is located on top of the foot.
- The foot is cleaned softly by absolute ethanol and dorsal vein is punctured with the needle of 23 G to 27 G. Drops of blood which appears on skin surface are collected in a capillary tube and after that little pressure is applied to stop the bleeding.

### Advantages:

- Pain and stress is less in this method

### Disadvantages:

- The volume of blood collected is not more.
- Frequent blood withdrawal is not possible.

## 1. Cardiac Puncture or Heart Puncture:

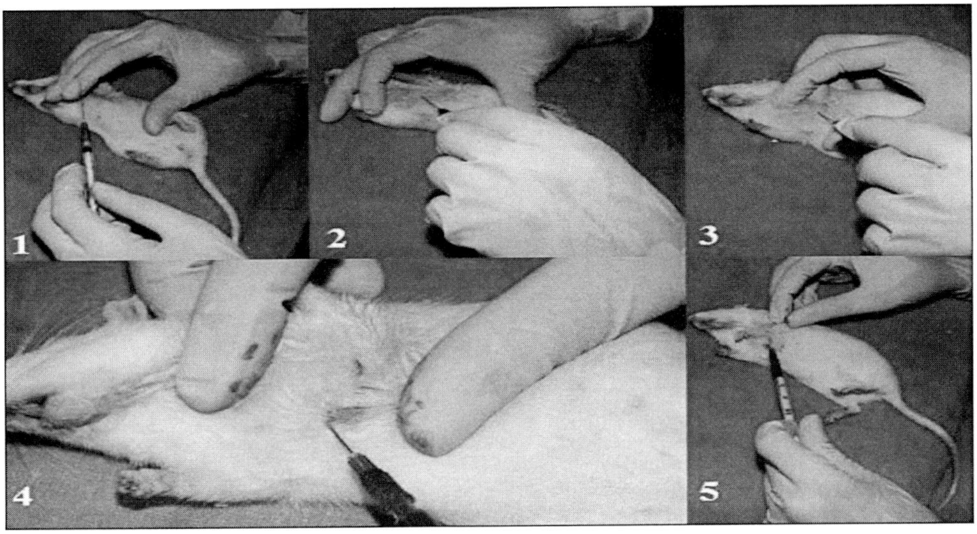


**Blood collection from the cardiac puncture or heart puncture**

### Procedure:

- Cardiac puncture has to be carried out in rat, mice and rabbit. This method is fully recommended for the animal having the terminal stage of the study to collect the large volume of blood from experimental animals.
- During the blood withdrawal from animals the animal will be in terminal anaesthesia.
- The needle (20-25G) is used for blood withdrawal with or without thoracotomy.
- Blood sample is collected from ventricles of the heart to avoid any collapse of heart.

### Advantages:

- Large volume of blood is collected.

### Disadvantage:

- Skillful person is needed.

## 2. Posterior vena cava:

### Procedure:

- In general, posterior vena cava blood sample is recommended for terminal stage of the study.

- Animal have to be anesthetized and 'Y'- or 'V'-shaped cut in the abdomen is made and the intestines are gently removed.
- The liver is pushed forward and the posterior vena cava (between the kidneys) is identified.
- 21 to 25G needle is inserted to collect blood from the posterior vena cava.
- This procedure will be repeated three to four times to collect more volume of blood sample.

## Summary of Blood Sampling Techniques:

| Route | Anesthesia Required | | Speed | | Sample Quality | | Repeat Samples | | Relative Obtainable Volume *(approximations)* | | Potential for Complications | |
|---|---|---|---|---|---|---|---|---|---|---|---|---|
| | Mouse | Rat | Mouse | Rat | Mouse | Rat | Mouse | Rat | Mouse | Rat | Mouse | Rat |
| **Tail Vein** | No | No | Med | Med | Fair | Good | Yes | Yes | Small *(50 ul)* | Small *(.2 mls)* | Low | Low |
| **Tail Artery** | No | No | Fast | Fast | Good | Very Good | Yes | Very Good | Medium *(100 ul)* | Medium *(.4 mls)* | Low | Low |
| **Retro-orbital** | No | Yes | Fast | Med | Very Good | Good | Alternate eyes | Alternate eyes | Med.-Large *(200 ul)* | Med.-Large *(.5 mls)* | Moderate -High | Moderate -High |
| **Saphenous** | No | No | Med. | Med | Good | Good | Yes | Yes | Small-Med. *(100 ul)* | Small-Med. *(.4 mls)* | Low | Low |
| **Mandibular Vein** | No | No | Slow-Med. | Slow-Med. | Fair-Good | Fair-Good | Yes | Yes | Small-Med. *(100 ul)* | Small-Med. *(.4 mls)* | Moderate | Moderate |
| **Mandibular Artery** | No | No | Very Fast | Very Fast | Very Good | Very Good | Yes | Yes | Large *(200 ul)* | Large *(.5 mls)* | Moderate | Moderate |

## Separate serum and plasma from blood:

Serum is the liquid fraction of whole blood that is collected after the blood is allowed to clot. The clot is removed by centrifugation and the resulting supernatant, designated serum, is carefully removed using a Pasteur pipette. Plasma is produced when whole blood is collected in tubes that are treated with an anticoagulant. The blood does not clot in the plasma tube. The cells are removed by centrifugation. The supernatant, designated plasma is carefully removed from the cell pellet using a Pasteur pipette.

## Serum preparation:

- Collect whole blood in a covered test tube. If commercially available tubes are to be used, the researcher should use the red topped tubes.
- These are available from Becton Dickinson (BD). BD's trade name for the blood handling tubes is Vacutainer.
- After collection of the whole blood, allow the blood to clot by leaving it undisturbed at room temperature.
- This usually takes 15–30 minutes. Remove the clot by centrifuging at 1,000–2,000 x g for 10 minutes in a refrigerated centrifuge.
- The resulting supernatant is designated serum. Following centrifugation, it is important to immediately transfer the liquid component (serum) into a clean polypropylene tube using a Pasteur pipette.
- The samples should be maintained at 2–8°C while handling. If the serum is not analyzed immediately, the serum should be apportioned into 0.5 ml aliquots, stored, and transported at –20°C or lower.
- It is important to avoid freeze-thaw cycles because this is detrimental to many serum components.
- Samples which are hemolyzed, icteric or lipemic can invalidate certain tests.

## Plasma preparation:

- Collect whole blood into commercially available anticoagulant-treated tubes e.g., EDTA-treated (lavender tops) or citrate-treated (light blue tops).
- Heparinized tubes (green tops) are indicated for some applications; however, heparin can often be contaminated with endotoxin, which can stimulate white blood cells to release cytokines.
- Cells are removed from plasma by centrifugation for 10 minutes at 1,000–2,000 x g using a refrigerated centrifuge. Centrifugation for 15 minutes at 2,000 x g depletes platelets in the plasma sample.
- The resulting supernatant is designated plasma.
- Following centrifugation, it is important to immediately transfer the liquid component (plasma) into a clean polypropylene tube using a Pasteur pipette.
- The samples should be maintained at 2–8°C while handling. If the plasma is not analyzed immediately, the plasma should be apportioned into 0.5 ml aliquots, stored, and transported at –20°C or lower.
- It is important to avoid freeze-thaw cycles. Samples which are hemolyzed, icteric, or lipemic can invalidate certain tests. There are other commercially available tubes for blood sample collection. Invitrogen has not evaluated some of these tubes for compatibility with our ELISA kits.

## Serum and plasma tubes:

| The commercially available serum tubes are as follows: | |
|---|---|
| Red | No anticoagulant. |
| Red with black | Treated with gel to help to separate the clot (not evaluated). |
| **The commercially available plasma tubes are as follows:** | |
| Lavender | Treated with EDTA. |
| Blue | Treated with citrate. |
| Green | Treated with heparin. |
| Grey | Treated with potassium oxalate/sodium fluoride (not evaluated). |
| Yellow | Treated with potassium oxalate/sodium fluoride (not evaluated). |

## Anaesthetics and Euthanasia used for animal studies:

A fundamental responsibility of individuals that use animals in research, teaching or testing is to anticipate and eliminate or minimize any potential that procedures may cause animal pain, distress, or discomfort.

Although animals that are in pain may not behave like humans, (e.g., pain in animals may be accompanied by immobility and silence, in contrast to the groans and cries of human patients), it is assumed that procedures that cause pain in humans cause pain in animals.

The presence of pain in animals can be recognized by alterations in animal behavior (e.g., reduced activity, reduced grooming, hunched- up posture, altered gait, changes in temperament, vocalizations, reduced food and water intake, reduced urinary and fecal output), and in physiological variables, (e.g., reduced depth of respiration, increased heart rate, and reduced hydration status).

Animal pain, distress, and discomfort can produce a range of undesirable physiological changes, which may radically alter measured responses to experimental stimuli, as well as the rate of recovery from surgical procedures, hence, its avoidance and alleviation are in the best interest of both the animal and researcher. Reducing post-procedural/post-operative pain, distress, and discomfort is accomplished by good nursing care, (e.g., keeping the animal warm, clean, dry and well padded), and by the administration of analgesic drugs.

In addition to the avoidance and alleviation of pain and discomfort, adequate post-procedural postoperative animal care also includes efforts to prevent and/or treat post-anesthetic complications, (e.g., aspiration, hypostatic pneumonia, cardiovascular and respiratory depression, dehydration, and infection). The prevention or minimization of animal pain, distress, or discomfort by the proper use of tranquilizers, anesthetics, and analgesics is scientifically and ethically essential to the humane care, use, and treatment of research animals.

## 1. Anaesthesia:

The word anaesthesia has been derived from Greek word that means "without perception of insensibility". Anesthesia is the act of providing sensation-free relief from pain or pain-producing procedures. Anesthesia must be performed by a person with knowledge of and familiarity with the drugs to be used in the animal species under consideration. There are numerous anesthetics available for use in rodents. Some of the more popular agents include:

a. **Chloralose**
b. **Urethane**
c. **Barbiturates**
d. **Paraldehyde**
e. **Magnesium Sulphate**
f. **Ketamine**
g. **Tribromoethanol**

### a. Chloralose:

- It is a compound of chloral and glucose prepared by heating equal parts of anhydrous glucose and charcoal, when both α- chloralose (active form) and β- chloralose (in active form) are formed.
- It is prepared as one percent solution by boiling in 0.9% NaCl or in distilled water, and administered intravenously or intraperitoneally at a temperature of 30-400°C before the chloralose comes out of solution.

**Disadvantages:** It is suitable only for acute experiments, usually in dogs and cats, inducing surgical anaesthesia for 3-4 hours or longer.

**Advantages:** It has the advantage of greater constancy of the depth of anaesthesia. The respiration and circulation are not depressed, and the blood pressure is well maintained usually on the higher side. Reflexes are not depressed but may be slightly exaggerated including responses to bilateral carotid occlusion.

### b. Urethane (Ethyl Carbamate):

- It is readily soluble in water giving a neutral solution. Usually 25% solution in water is used.

**Disadvantages:** It is suitable only for acute experiments since it has delayed toxic effect on liver, and may also cause agranulocytosis and pulmonary adenomata. Mice develop an exceptionally high incidence of lung tumors regardless of the route of administration.

### c. Barbiturates:

- Barbiturates interfere with nerve impulse transmission both in the central nervous system and in the ganglia producing depression of cardiovascular and spinal cord reflexes.
- In rabbits pedal reflex (leg retraction) is lost first, then pupillary and finally palpebral reflex.
- Pentobarbital is a barbiturate and, historically, the most commonly used anesthetic in rodents.

**Advantages:** At recommended doses, it causes minimal cardiovascular depression. It is also relatively long acting and can provide approximately 45 minutes of surgical anesthesia.

**Disadvantages:** Pentobarbital is a potent inducer of the hepatic microsomal enzyme system. Causes pronounced respiratory depression as well as hypothermia, particularly when repeated doses are given. Phenobarbitone sodium and barbitone sodium are used for prolonged experiments. Thiopentone sodium (pentothal) is used for surgical operations of short duration. It produces rapid induction with minimum excitation.

### d. Paraldehyde:

**Advantages:** It has a wide margin of safety because it depresses only the cerebrum and not the medullary centres. Intravenous injection is likely to produce cardiac dilatation and pulmonary congestion and oedema.

**Disadvantages:** Under its influence the basal blood pressure as well as the response to vasopressor and depressor drugs are low. Bilateral carotid occlusion produces poor pressor response or even a depressor response.

### e. Magnesium Sulphate:

- A 20% magnesium sulphate solution 5ml/kg intravenously produces anaesthesia for about an hour. Calcium gluconate intravenously will counteract its depressant effect immediately. Its principal use is in producing euthanasia.

### f. Tribromoethanol:

**Advantages:** In most rodents, tribromoethanol produces good surgical anesthesia, with good skeletal muscle relaxation and only a moderate degree of respiratory depression. It is relatively inexpensive and not a controlled agent.

**Disadvantages:** It is potential for causing peritonitis. When exposed to either light or temperatures >400C, tribromoethanol degrades into two byproducts: hydrobromic acid and dibromo acetaldehyde. Both of these compounds are highly irritating when administered IP and result in peritonitis and visceral adhesions which may be fatal.

### g. Ketamine Hydrochloride:

Ketamine hydrochloride, a dissociative anesthetic, disrupts pain transmission and suppresses spinal cord activity with some action at opioid receptors. Visceral pain is not abolished with dissociative anesthetics and there is poor muscle relaxation and analgesia.

**Disadvantages:** Ketamine is a poor anesthetic when used alone, but is more often combined with other agents. When combined with other drugs, it is usually administered IP. Ketamine is acidic, can be irritating, and cause muscle necrosis when administrated IM. Ketamine-induced nerve damage can cause self mutilation in rodents. Ketamine is a controlled substance. Store in a locked cabinet and maintain a log of its use.

## 2. Euthanasia:

The term euthanasia is derived from the Greek terms eu meaning good and thanatos meaning death. The act of inducing humane death in an animal by a method that induces rapid loss of consciousness and death with a minimum of pain, discomfort or distress. Methods of euthanasia fall into two broad categories:

### Chemical methods:

#### Inhalant agents:

Eg.: Ether, Halothane, Methoxyflurane, Isoflurane, Enflurane, Chloroform, Nitrogen, Nitrous oxide, Carbon dioxide, Carbon monoxide, Argon, Hydrogen cyanide.

#### Injectable agents:

Eg: Barbiturates, Chloral hydrate, Ethanol, Ketamine, Magnesium sulphate, Potassium chloride, Neuromuscular blocking agents.

### Physical methods:

Eg.: Penetrating Captive Bolt, Euthanasia by a Blow to the Head, Gunshot, Cervical Dislocatiod, Decapitation, Electrocution, Microwave Irradiation, Thoracic (Cardiopulmonary, Cardiac) Compression, Kill Traps, Maceration, Adjunctive Methods, Exsanguination, Stunning, Pithing.

## Introduction about some common methods of euthanasia:

- **Inhalation of anesthesia gas** – acceptable with conditions for rodents and other small animals (< 7 kg). Typically used as part of a two-step process with a secondary physical method of euthanasia such as decapitation or cervical dislocation.
- **Inhalation of $CO_2$** - acceptable with conditions, including the special considerations listed below.
- **Immersion agents** – e.g. MS 222/Tricaine. Acceptable for aquatic species, usually in connection with a secondary physical method.
- **Cervical Dislocation** – acceptable for small birds, mice and immature rats. Requires training and should be performed under anesthesia unless specifically approved by the CPCSEA.
- **Decapitation** – acceptable for rodents and small rabbits. Requires training; anesthesia recommended unless approved by the CPCSEA. Guillotines must be sharpened and adjusted frequently to ensure proper performance.
- **Injectable barbiturate agents** – e.g. sodium pentobarbital, Euthasol®, Eutha 6®, Fatal Plus® - acceptable for most species.
- **Exsanguination/Cardiac Perfusion** – acceptable with conditions; animals must be anesthetized.

## Special considerations for the use of carbon dioxide gas as a euthanasia agent:

The following additional guidelines must be followed when using $CO_2$:

- $CO_2$ must be delivered from compressed gas canister only. Gas should be delivered using a gradual fill method- a displacement rate from 10% to 30% of the chamber volume per minute is recommended. Use of a flow meter is strongly recommended.
- Use of dry ice to deliver $CO_2$ gas is unacceptable.
- High concentrations of $CO_2$ have been determined to cause pain and distress. The practice of immersion, where conscious animals are placed directly into a container filled with 100% $CO_2$, is unacceptable.
- Use of the rodents' home cage is recommended as it minimizes stress in the animals.
- Chambers used for $CO_2$ euthanasia must not be overcrowded. Overcrowding in this situation is defined as less than one half the normal housing space normally required for the animals.
- If animals are removed from their home cages prior to euthanasia, the container used to transport animals between the housing area and procedure room/euthanasia chamber must not be overcrowded.
- Male mice from different cages should not be mixed in transport cages or the euthanasia chamber to prevent distress and/or fighting.

- Detailed instructions for the use of CO2 euthanasia are posted in all vivarium procedure rooms and can be reviewed on the CPCSEA website.

## VIVA-VOCE

**Q.1 Write down the principle of Blood collection Process.**

**Ans: Principle:**

- The collection process of blood sample should be less painful and stressful.
- If the experiments need multiple collection of blood then rabbit can be used.
- About 10% of total circulating blood volume can be withdrawn from healthy, normal, adult animal without causing considerable changes in its physiology and the animal should not bleed for 3 weeks at least in single withdrawn.
- If the blood collection exceeds 10% of total volume of blood then fluid replacement may be required. The special care should be taken for pregnant, obese and older animals.

**Q.2 Write down the full form of IAEC.**

**Ans:** Institute of Animal Ethics Committee.

**Q.3 Define Anaesthesia.**

**Ans:** The word anaesthesia has been derived from Greek word that means "without perception of insensibility". Anesthesia is the act of providing sensation-free relief from pain or pain-producing procedures.

**Q.4 Write down the methods of euthanasia.**

**Ans: Some common methods of euthanasia:**

- Inhalation of anesthesia gas
- Inhalation of CO2
- Immersion agents
- Cervical Dislocation
- Decapitation
- Injectable barbiturate agents
- Exsanguination/Cardiac Perfusion

# Experiment No. 6

## Object: To study the different routes of drugs administration in mice/rats.

## Introduction:

The route of administration is largely dependent on the property of the test substance and the objective of the experiment. All administration should be performed with knowledge of the chemical and physical characteristics of the substance. All routes have both demerit and merit, such as the absorption, bioavailability and metabolism of the substance. Consideration should be paid to the pH, viscosity, concentration, sterility, pyrogenicity, toxicity as well as the existence of hazardous substances. A knowledge of available methods and techniques of administration as well as knowledge of the deposition and fate of the administered substance will help the scientist/ investigator to select the most appropriate route for her/his purpose. This route must be selected before the start of any experiment.

Proper restraint is the most important technique when animal were treated as this decreases stress and increases successful treatment. Personnel using experimental animals should be well trained in handling and restraint, should obtain authentication for responsible use of experimental animals and attain a scientifically high standard. Further experience will lead to repeatable and reliable results. During administration animal should be protected from pain, suffering, distress or lasting harm or at least pain and distress shall be kept to a minimum. Some injections (such as footpad injection) are strongly discouraged and if required must be justified on a case by case basis.

## Principles of administration:

**Handling and restraint:** Good handling and restraint is the most important technique for correct administration. Proper restraining leads to successful administration and varies with the routes of administration. Disposable gloves must be worn as manual restraint is frequently used for injections. There are two styles of manual restraint, one uses both hands and the other is single handed.

## Double handed manual restraint:

- The mouse is lifted by the base of the tail and placed on the cage lid or other solid surface with one hand and then its tail is pulled gently back.

- It is quickly and firmly picked up by the scruff of the neck behind the ears with the thumb and index finger of the other hand.
- The tail is transferred from the first hand to between the palm and little or ring finger of the other hand, then fixed. The mouse is restrained.

## Single handed restraint:

- The tail is picked up using thumb and fore finger of the chosen hand, then the mouse is placed on the cage lid or other solid surface.
- The tail is immediately grasped by the palm and middle finger, ring finger and/or little finger, and the thumb and forefinger released.
- The fold of skin from the scruff of neck down the back is immediately gripped using the thumb and forefinger. The mouse is then restrained.
- To prevent kicking by the hind legs, the tail is fixed using the palm and forefinger and then the left hind leg is held firmly between the ring and little finger (where the mouse is restrained by the left hand

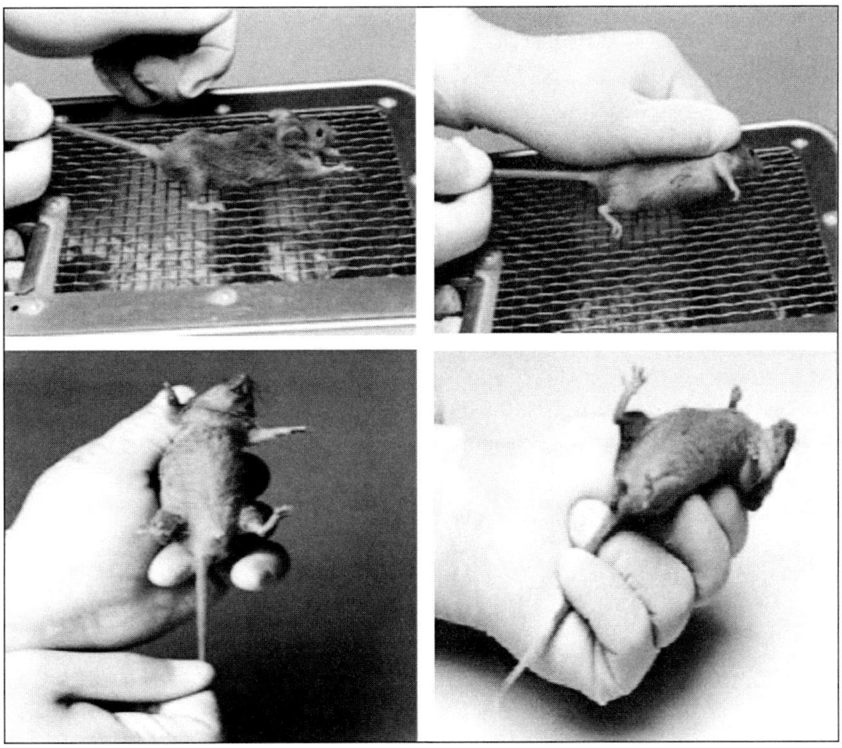

**Manual restraint of a mouse using both hands. (a)** The mouse is placed on the cage lid with the preferred hand. The tail is pulled gently back by the hand. **(b)** The mouse is quickly and firmly picked up by the scruff of the neck behind the ears with thumb and index finger of other hand. **(c)** The tail is transferred from the preferred hand to between palm and little or ring finger of the other hand, then held firmly. **(d)** The mouse is restrained.

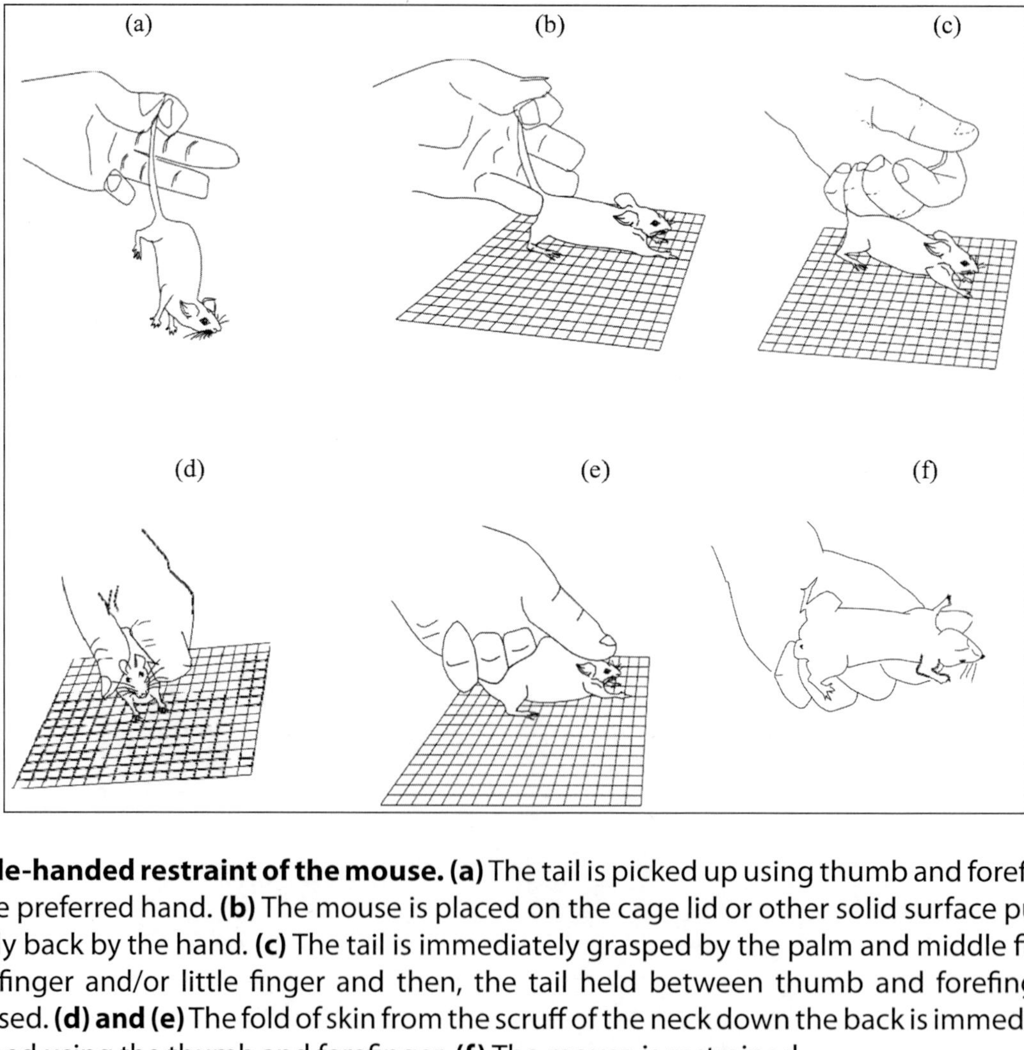


**Single-handed restraint of the mouse. (a)** The tail is picked up using thumb and forefinger of the preferred hand. **(b)** The mouse is placed on the cage lid or other solid surface pulling gently back by the hand. **(c)** The tail is immediately grasped by the palm and middle finger, ring finger and/or little finger and then, the tail held between thumb and forefinger is released. **(d) and (e)** The fold of skin from the scruff of the neck down the back is immediately gripped using the thumb and forefinger. **(f)** The mouse is restrained.

## Preparation of the site:

The area for administration is clipped or cleaned with warm water if necessary before cleaning the skin is treated with alcohol- or disinfectant-moistened cotton. Where aseptic skin is necessary; the fur must be clipped followed by a three-stage surgical preparation:

surgical soap, alcoholic rinse and surgical preparation solution. The skin is dried immediately before administration. In some cases a local anesthetic may be applied first to prevent pain.

## I. Enteral administration:

Enteral administration has the advantages that it is possible to give quite large amounts of non-sterile sub- stances or solution and that a pH as low as 3 can be administrated by this route. On the other hand, alkaline solutions are very poorly tolerated by mouth. When using the oral route it should be under- stood that substances can be destroyed by the gastric juices and that the food content of the stomach influences both rate and order of the gastric emptying. The rate of absorption is markedly influenced by its time of residence in the stomach and is also directly related to the rate at which substances are passed from the stomach into the intestine. Enzymes of the host and microflora of the digestive tract can also metabolize the substance. On the other hand some insoluble substances become solubilized as the result of enzymatic activity during their passage through the stomach and intestine making absorption possible. The two major methods for enteral administration are mixing the substance with food or water or direct administration using gavage. Rectal administration is also possible.

### Oral administration:

The simplest method for administration is to give the substance with food or drinking water. However, this is not practicable with those that are unpalatable, insoluble or chemically unstable in drinking water or when they irritate the mucosa of the gastrointestinal tract. The daily food and water intake of mouse should be known before the experiment, to calculate the quantity of substance to be mixed.

Because food and water wastage happens all the time, it is difficult to determine the precise amount of food and water intake and therefore the precise intake of the substance. The only way this can be done is by keeping mice in metabolic cages and recording the wastage.

### Intragastric administration:

Direct administration by oral gavage is preferred to mixing substances with food or drinking water because the intake of the substances is precisely measured. A ball tip needle is used to prevent damaging the oesophagus and from passing through the glottal opening into the trachea. A 22 G ball tip needle is suit- able for administration to adult mice. The conscious mouse is manually restrained firmly by gripping a fold of skin from the scruff of neck down the back, immobilization of the head is essential for this procedure. When the neck is extended the position is vertical. A straight line is formed between the mouth and the cardiac sphincter through the oesophageal orifice. The needle is passed gently through the mouth and pharynx into the oesophagus.

The mouse usually swallows as the feeding needle approaches the pharynx, these swallowing movements can help so that the probe slips through the oesophageal opening. The substance is then administered slowly. If any obstruction is felt, if the mouse coughs, chokes or begins to struggle vigorously after the gavage begins, or if fluid is seen coming out through the nose, these may indicate that the needle has entered the lungs. Any of these signs would necessitate immediate withdrawal of the needle, and the mouse must be observed very carefully. If there is any sign that fluid has got into the lungs, the mouse should be euthanized. As soon as administration is finished, the needle must be withdrawn. A volume of >2 ml is recommended.

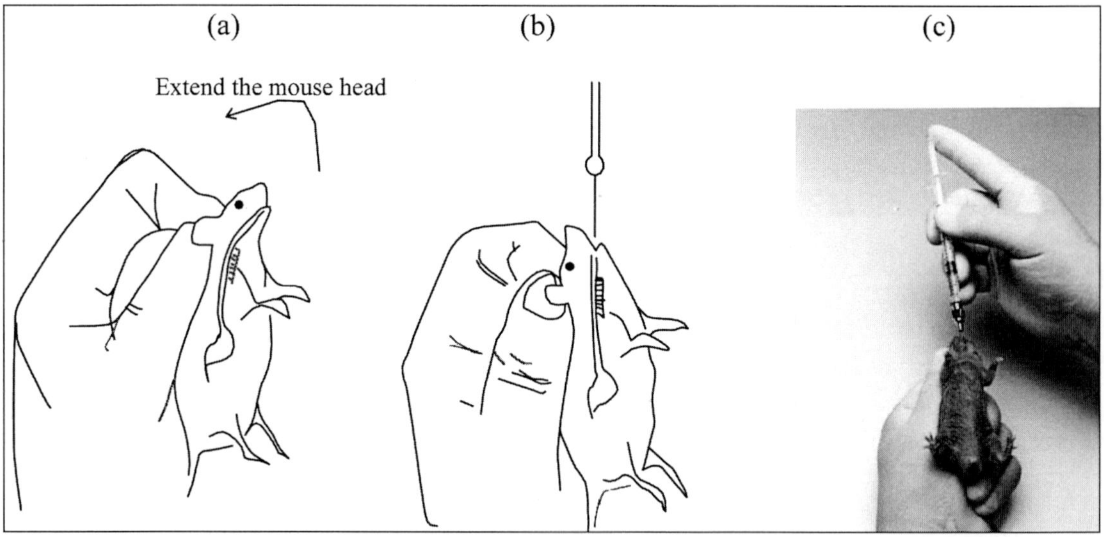


**Procedure for intragastric administration using a ball tip needle. (a)** First extend the neck; **(b)** A straight line is formed between the mouth and stomach; **(c)** Intragastric injection using 1.0 ml syringe with 22 G × 1.0 in. feeding needle is made.

## II. Parenteral administration:

Administration of substances other than via the alimentary canal to the body includes injection, infusion, topical application and inhalation, and implantation of an osmotic pump or a controlled-release drug delivery pellet. Small amounts of solution are injected, and large volumes are infused. In both cases the skin must be penetrated by a needle.

## 1. Subcutaneous administration (s.c.):

Subcutaneous administrations are easy. As they are rarely painful a conscious mouse can usually be used. The rate of absorption is lower than from intraperitoneal or intramuscular injections.

Subcutaneous administrations are made into the loose skin over the interscapular or inguinal area. Subcutaneous administrations over the interscapular area are made as follows. The mouse is manually restrained and then placed on a clean towel or solid surface. The needle is inserted under the skin of the interscapular area tented by the thumb and forefinger and the substance then injected. A volume <3 ml is recommended. Subcutaneous administration over the inguinal area is made as follows. The mouse is restrained manually and the head tilted downwards. Holding the hind leg firmly helps this procedure. The needle is inserted into the lower left or right quadrant of abdomen avoiding the abdominal midline and the substance injected. A volume of <0.2 ml/site is recommended. To mini- mize leakage, the needle should be advanced several millimeters through the subcutaneous tissue.

**(A)** **(B)**

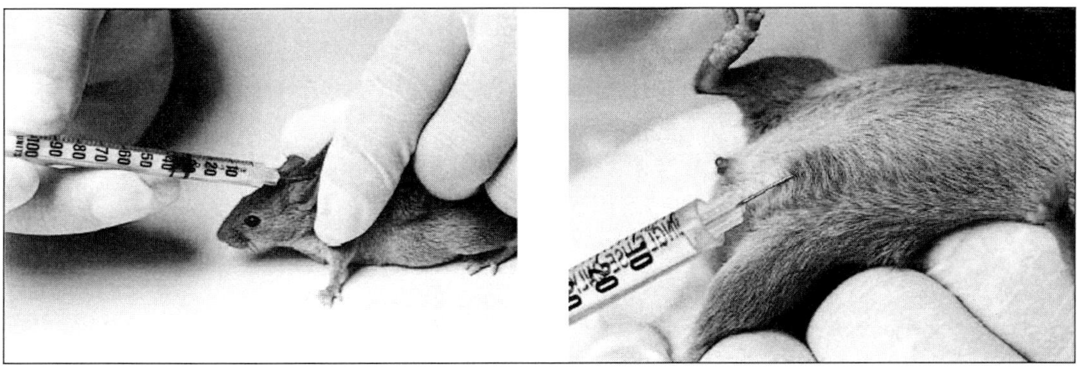

**Subcutaneous injection.** **(a)** Subcutaneous injection at the base of a fold of loose skin (area at the neck) using an Insulin syringe: 27 G × 1/2 in., 1.0 ml; **(b)** subcutaneous injection at the lower left quadrant using an Insulin syringe: 27 G × 1/2 in., 1.0 ml.

## 2. Intraperitoneal administration (i.p.):

This is the most common route being technically simple and easy. It allows quite long periods of absorption from the repository site. The rate of absorption by this route is usually one-half to one-fourth as rapid as from the intravenous one. Limitations are the sensitivity of the tissue to irritating substances, less tolerance to solutions of non-physiological pH. These should be isotonic and quite large volume can be administered by this route.

The conscious mouse is manually restrained and is held in a supine position with its posterior end slightly elevated or the head can be tilted lower than the body. The needle and syringe should be kept almost parallel to its vertebral column in order to avoid accidental penetration of the viscera. The needle is pushed in at an approximately 10° angle between the needle and the abdominal surface in the lower quadrant of the abdomen. To avoid leakage from the puncture point, the needle is run through subcutaneous tissue in a cranial direction for 2–3 mm and then inserted through the abdominal wall. The recommended volume is >3.0 ml.

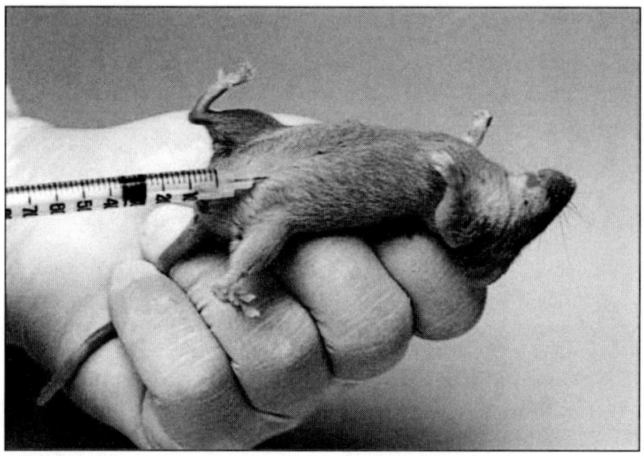

**Intraperitoneal injection to lower left quadrant using an Insulin syringe: 27 G × 1/2 in., 1.0 ml.**

### 3. Intravenous administration (i.v.):

Intravenous injection has advantages over other routes. Solutions at a high concentration, high or low pH or irritating can be administered intravenously provided that the rate of injection is kept slow and precautions are taken to avoid getting the solution outside the vein. Compounds that are poorly absorbed by the digestive tract may be given intravenously but intravenous administrations require technical expertise and skill. The syringe plus needle or the catheter must first be filled with the solution to remove air bubbles. Administrations are usually made into the lateral tail veins not into the dorsal tail vein, as it is not straight. The lateral veins are readily visualized, but have quite small diameters. If anaesthesia is not used, a restraining device is usually necessary.

The mouse is either placed in the restrainer or anesthetized and the tail is then warmed with a lamp or warm towel, or immersed in warm water (40–45°C) in order to dilate the vessels. The tail is swabbed with 70% alcohol on a gauze sponge or swab. Insert the needle parallel to the tail vein penetrating 2–4 mm into the lumen while keeping the bevel of the needle face upwards. The solution is then injected slowly and no resistance should be felt if the solution is properly administered. The injected solution temporarily replaces the blood but then should be washed away by the blood stream. If this does not happen the position of the needle is certainly not in the vein but in the surrounding tissue so it must be moved in the surrounding tissue in such a way that it then enters the vein or a new try must be made. When the intravenous administration is finished or the cannula is pulled out, the injection site must be pressed firmly with a swab or fingers to prevent backflow of the administered solution and/or blood. If the same vein must be used several times the first administration should be made as distal as possible in relation to the heart and subsequent administrations should be placed progressively more proximally. Because venipuncture and the administration of substances can damage and/or block the vein, the distal part of vein may no longer be used. The recommended volume is <0.2 ml.

The ophthalmic plexus route is also used for intravenous administration. The technique resembles the blood collection by retro- orbital sinus puncture. The mouse is anesthetized, and then manually restrained on a solid surface being held gently but firmly by the nape of the neck. By pressing down with the thumb and forefinger in the occipital area and pulling back the skin, the point of the needle can be directed toward the back of the orbit at a 20–40° angle. The needle is inserted medially through the conjunctiva on the inner side of the ocular cavity. If entry is blocked by bone, the needle is withdrawn slightly. Fluid is injected slowly loosening the skin slightly. Also this route is useful for rescuing mice showing anaphylaxis by administration of an isotonic solution.

Other routes for intravenous administration via the external jugular vein, the dorsal metatarsal vein and the sublingual vein have been reported.

(a) (b)

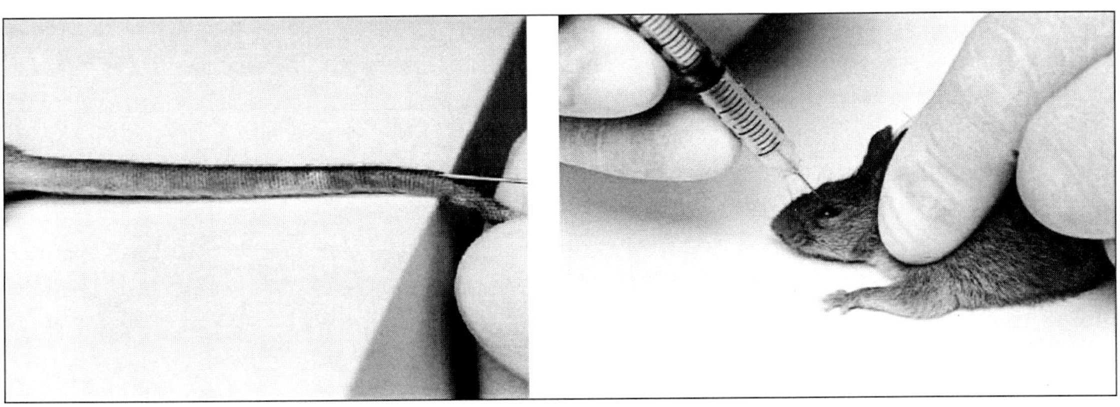

**(a)** intravenous injection into the lateral tail vein of an anesthetized mouse using an Insulin syringe: 27 G × 1/2 in., 1.0 ml.

**(b)** intravenous injection into the retro- orbital sinus of an anesthetized mouse using an Insulin syringe: 27 G × 1/2 in., 1.0 ml.

### 4. Intramuscular administration (i.m.):

This should usually be avoided, as mouse muscles are small. If necessary, it may be given into the thigh muscle with injection volumes <0.05 ml. The tip of needle should be directed away from the femur and sciatic nerve. The mouse is anesthetized or is manually restrained by another person. The needle tip is inserted through the skin and into the muscle. Aspirate briefly with the syringe before injection. If blood or body fluid reverses, stop the procedure. The needle must be moved or a fresh attempt must be made. Good technique and restraint are necessary and intramuscular administration should only be performed by well-trained personnel.

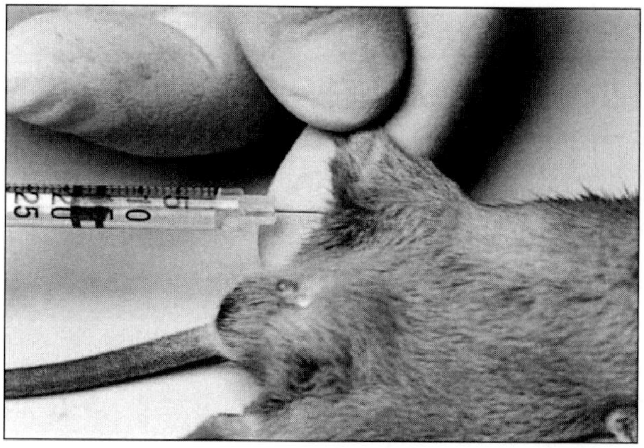

**Intramuscular injection into the leg muscle**

### 5. Intradermal administration:

It is very difficult in the mouse due to the very thin skin. Using a fine needle (29 G or smaller) is recommended. The mouse is anesthetized, the fur clipped or hair removed from an area on the back, ventral abdomen, or hind footpad, which is wiped with 70% ethanol on a gauze sponge or swab. The skin is held tautly with thumb and index finger and the needle inserted, bevel up and at a shallow angle, just under the superficial layer of epidermis. The volume should be <0.05 ml per site. Resistance should be felt both as the needle is advanced and as the compound is injected. A hard bleb will be seen upon successful intradermal injection of even a small quantity of fluid. If multiple sites are injected, adequate separation is necessary to prevent coalescing of lesions.

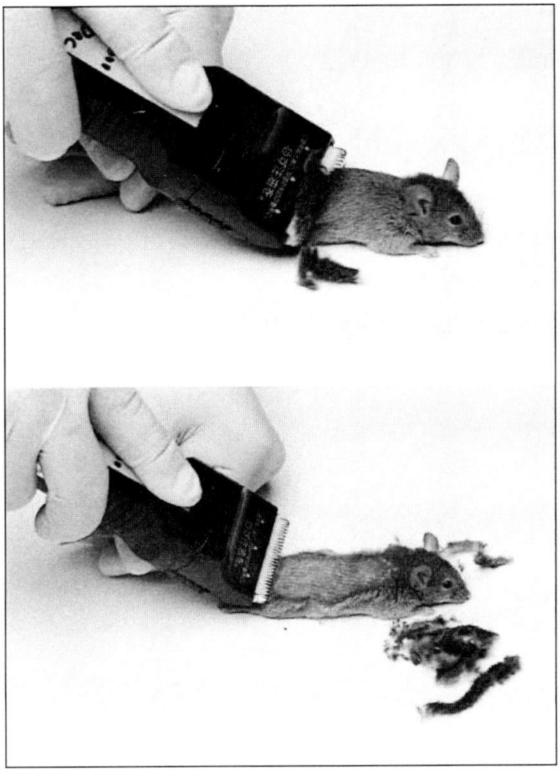

**Clipping of hair on the back. Hair on the back is clipped by a cordless electric clipper**

## IV. Inhalation:

The inhalation route incidentally is the nearest akin to an intravenous injection because of the relatively large area presented for absorption by a membrane that is separated from the blood by only one or two cell layers. Consequently, absorption of gases and aerosols that reach the alveoli is virtually complete. The greatest problems surrounding the use of the inhalation route are the generation of a suitable aerosol of the test substance, if it is not sufficiently volatile, a constant and suitable air level of the material under study and the determination of the dosage given. Both small and large particle sizes are not adequate, it is generally believed that particle size of 0.5–2.0 μm in diameter are optimum.

## V. Implantable pump, controlled- release drug delivery pellet and cannulas:

The delivery of substances at a slow, steady rate over period of days, weeks or months without the need for external connection or frequent animal handling can be supplied by using an osmotic pump or controlled- release drug delivery pellets.

Osmotic pumps, ALZET pump, can be used for systemic administration when implanted subcutaneously or intraperitoneally or can be attached to a catheter for intravenous, intracerebral or intra-arterial infusion. The pumps have been used to target delivery to a wide variety of sites including the spinal cord, spleen, liver, organ or tissue transplants and wound healing sites.

Controlled-release drug delivery pellets effectively and continuously release the active product in the animal. The pellets are intended for, although not limited to, simple subcutaneous implantation in laboratory animals.

Implantable cannulas permit continuous access to the venous or arterial system for either intravenous substance administration or blood withdrawal. Using strict aseptic techniques, the cannula is inserted into a vein or artery (the femoral vessels, jugular vein, and carotid artery are common sites) and secured in place. The other end of the cannula is attached to a small port that is secured in a subcutaneous location, most often over the shoulders.

## VIVA-VOCE

**Q.1 Define double handed manual restraint.**

**Ans: Double handed manual restraint:**

- The mouse is lifted by the base of the tail and placed on the cage lid or other solid surface with one hand and then its tail is pulled gently back.
- It is quickly and firmly picked up by the scruff of the neck behind the ears with the thumb and index finger of the other hand.
- The tail is transferred from the first hand to between the palm and little or ring finger of the other hand, then fixed. The mouse is restrained.

**Q.2 Define single handed restraint.**

**Ans: Single handed restraint:**

- The tail is picked up using thumb and fore finger of the chosen hand, then the mouse is placed on the cage lid or other solid surface.
- The tail is immediately grasped by the palm and middle finger, ring finger and/or little finger, and the thumb and forefinger released.
- The fold of skin from the scruff of neck down the back is immediately gripped using the thumb and forefinger. The mouse is then restrained.
- To prevent kicking by the hind legs, the tail is fixed using the palm and forefinger and then the left hind leg is held firmly between the ring and little finger (where the mouse is restrained by the left hand)

# Experiment No. 7

## Object: To study the effect of hepatic microsomal enzyme inducers on the phenobarbitone sleeping time in mice.

## Principle:

The drugs which induce hepatic microsomal oxidative enzyme system enhance the metabolism of other drugs. As a result in the presence of an enzyme-inducer the duration of action of second drug will be reduced. This has significant clinical relevance because when more than one drug is administered at a time one drug may modify the action of another through the microsomal enzyme inducing property.

The common drugs which induce hepatic microsomal enzyme system are phenobarbitone and meprobamate. Co-administration of any drug with either of these drugs may effect the disposition of the second drug and therefore, the desired pharmacological effects.

## Requirement:

**Animal:** Mice (20-25g)

**Drugs:** Phenobarbitone sodium (dose: 50mg/kg i.p), Pentobarbital sodium (dose: 45 mg/ml).

## Procedure:

1. Weigh and number the animals.
2. Divide them into two groups, each comprising of at least 6 mice.
3. To the first group inject phenobarbitone once daily for 5 days.
4. To the second group inject distilled water, similarly, for 5 days.
5. One hour after the last dose of phenobarbitone on the 5$^{th}$ day, inject pentobarbital to both the groups.
6. Note the onset and duration of sleep due to pentobarbital in both the groups.

## Observation table:

| S.No. | Body wt.(g) | Treatment | Dose (mg/kg) | Onset of action (min.) | Duration of action (min.) | %reduction in sleeptime |
|---|---|---|---|---|---|---|
| 1. | | Pentobarbital | | | | |
| 2. | | | | | | |
| 3 | | | | | | |
| 4. | | | | | | |
| 5. | | | | | | |
| Mean | | | | | | |
| 1. | | Phenobarbitone + Pentobarbital | | | | |
| 2. | | | | | | |
| 3. | | | | | | |
| 4. | | | | | | |
| 5. | | | | | | |
| Mean | | | | | | |

## Precautions:

1. Handle the animals with care.
2. Maintain the laboratory conditions properly.

# VIVA-VOCE

**Q.1 Write down the principle of hepatic microsomal enzyme inducers on the phenobarbitone sleeping time in mice.**

**Ans:** The drugs which induce hepatic microsomal oxidative enzyme system enhance the metabolism of other drugs. As a result in the presence of an enzyme-inducer the duration of action of second drug will be reduced. This has significant clinical relevance because when more than one drug is administered at a time one drug may modify the action of another through the microsomal enzyme inducing property.

The common drugs which induce hepatic microsomal enzyme system are phenobarbitone and meprobamate. Co-administration of any drug with either of these drugs may effect the disposition of the second drug and therefore, the desired pharmacological effects. The students are advised to study various processes of drug metabolism before doing this experiment.

# Experiment No. 8

## Object: To study the effect of drugs on ciliary motility of frog oesophagus.

## Principles:

Cilia are thin hair like structures present in the ciliated epithelium cells, found in the respiratory tract, digestive tract, fallopian tube and central canal of spinal cord. The buccal cavity and oesophagus contains cilia which help in the movement of food particles. The ciliary motility in buccal cavity and oesophagus are stimulated by acetylcholine and other cholinergic drugs. On other hand, anti-cholinergic drugs like atropine paralyze the cilia and decrease ciliary motility.

**Parasympathomimetics:** This drug produces similar action like acetylcholine. They are also called as cholinomimetics. Ex. Bethanechol, Methacholine and Choline alkaloids like muscarine, pilocarpine.

**Anticholinesterases:** These are the agents which inhibit the cholinesterase enzyme and protect Ach from hydrolysis potentiate Ach action. Ex. Neostigmine, Pyridostigmine.

**Parasympatholytics:** These drugs prevent the action of Ach by blocking the muscarinic cholinergic receptors. They are also called as anticholinergic drugs. Ex. Atropine, Hyosine etc.

## Requirements:

**Animal:** Frog

**Drugs:** Physostigmine stock solution (1 µg/ml), Atropine stock solution (1 µg/ml)

**Physiological solution:** Normal saline

**Equipments:** Frog board, stop-watch and surgical instruments.

## Procedure:

1. Decapitate the frog and pin the frog to the frog board on its back.
2. Pin the lower jaw to the abdomen cutting sufficiently the buccal cavity and exposing the oesophagus. Keep the buccal cavity and the opening of the oesophagus wet by irrigating it with normal saline.

3. Fix two parts i.e. from a point in the lower jaw to the beginning of the oesophagus. Keep this distance constant to measure the time taken by the particle to move from a fixed point in the lower jaw to the beginning of the oesophagus.
4. Place a poppy seed or a small piece of cork at the remarked spot in jaw. Turn on the stop watch and note the time taken by the object to reach the beginning of the oesophagus. Repeat this several times.
5. Put a few drops of physostigmine on the buccal cavity and after 10 min repeat step 4, note the time.
6. Wash the buccal cavity with normal saline. Put a few drops of atropine on the buccal cavity. After 10 min repeat the step 4. Note the time.
7. Find out the differences in the time taken by the object to move between the pre-marked distance in the buccal cavity in presence of saline, physostigmine and atropine.

## Observation table:

| S.No. | Treatment | Approximate Distance (cm) | Observations (sec) | | | | |
|---|---|---|---|---|---|---|---|
| | | | 1 | 2 | 3 | 4 | 5 |
| 1 | Saline | | | | | | |
| 2 | | | | | | | |
| 3 | | | | | | | |
| 4 | | | | | | | |
| Mean | | | | | | | |
| 1 | Physostigmine | | | | | | |
| 2 | | | | | | | |
| 3 | | | | | | | |
| 4 | | | | | | | |
| Mean | | | | | | | |
| 1 | Atropine | | | | | | |
| 2 | | | | | | | |
| 3 | | | | | | | |
| 4 | | | | | | | |
| Mean | | | | | | | |

## Precautions:

1. Handle the animals with care.
2. Maintain the laboratory conditions properly.
3. Dissect the frog carefully.

## VIVA-VOCE

**Q.1 Define Parasympathomimetic.**

**Ans:** Parasympathomimetic drug produces similar action like acetylcholine. They are also called as cholinomimetics.

**Q.2 Define Parasympatholytics:**

**Ans:** These drugs prevent the action of Ach by blocking the muscarinic cholinergic receptors. They are also called as anticholinergic drugs.

**Q.3 Define Anticholinesterases:**

**Ans:** These are the agents which inhibit the cholinesterase enzyme and protect Ach from hydrolysis, potentiate Ach action.

# Experiment No. 9

## Object: To study the effect of drugs on rabbit eye.

## Principle:

There are various number of drugs that are used for their local action in the eye as eye ointments and eye drops. Most of these drugs belong to the class of autonomic or local anaesthetic, antimicrobial groups. The sphincter papillae of the iris have parasympathetic supply which exercise dominant control. The opposite effects are produced by the relaxation of ciliary muscle resulting in paralysis of accommodation. Topically applied drug can affect the eye by changing conjunctival congestion, papillary size, corneal sensitivity, light reflex and intraocular pressure. However the effect of drug on papillary size, light reflex and corneal reflex can be studied and observed by students easily. Cornea is more sensitive part of eye which respond to touch. When local anaesthetics are instilled in eye, it abolishes the corneal reflex by blocking the conduction of nerve.

Mydriatics are the drugs that dilate the pupils and miotics are the drug which constrict the pupil. Ephedrine (4%), atropine (1%), homatropine (0.5%), adrenaline (0.1%) used as mydriatics and pilocarpine (1-4%), physostigmine (1%) used as miotics in rabbits. Ephedrine causes the constriction of radial muscle of iris and dilate pupils, and pilocarpine constricts circular muscle of iris and causes miosis.

## Testing of reflexes:

1. **Corneal touch reflexes:** Can be studied by touching the cornea of eye with a cotton pledget or a piece of paper and observing whether the rabbit is blinking the eyelids or not. Check in both control eye and test eyes.
2. **Light reflexes:** it is studied by focusing a torch on the eye and observing whether the pupil is constricted in response to the light or not. Check in both control eye and test eye.
3. **Effects of drug on diameter of pupils:** the dilation or constriction of pupil after adding the drug solution is observed and compared with the diameter of pupil in both the eyes.

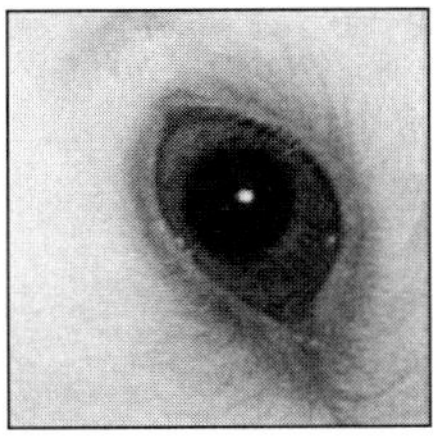

Pupil Dilate

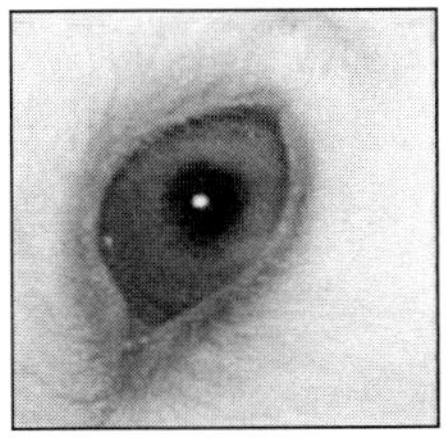

Constricted Pupil

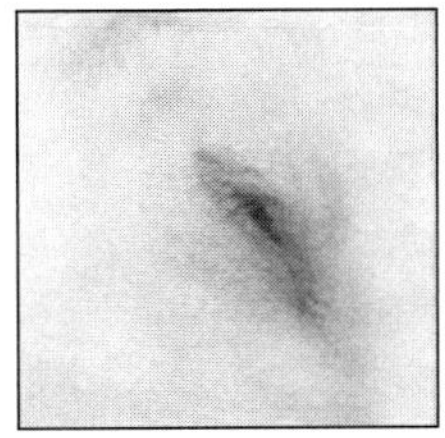

Blinking of eye

## A. local anaesthetic effect on rabbit eye:

### Requirement:

**Animal:** Rabbits (1.5-2.5 kg)

**Drugs:** Lignocaine (4% w/v) or atropine (1% w/v)

**Equipment:** Rabbit holder, dropper, cotton swab.

### Procedure:

1. Place the rabbit in the rabbit holder, by keeping the head outside the holder. Acclimatize the rabbit for 5 minute in rabbit holder.
2. Observe the size of the pupil in both the eyes
3. Prepare stock solution of lignocaine (4% w/v) or atropine (1% w/v).
4. Examine the effect of light reflex by holding the torch in front of the eye or stick the cotton swab on eye to see the reflex on both eye.
5. Instill few drops of either lignocaine or atropine solution using dropper in right eye of the rabbit.
6. The left eye would serve as control and instill few drops of normal saline.
7. Record corneal reflex before and after 2, 4, 6, 8, 10, 20 and 30 minute of drug instillation. Tabulate the observation as '+' for presence of corneal reflex and '-' for absence of corneal reflex.

### Observation table:

| Time (Min) | Corneal Reflex (Present/Absent) | |
|---|---|---|
| | Left Eye | Right Eye |
| 2 | | |
| 4 | | |
| 6 | | |
| 8 | | |
| 10 | | |
| 20 | | |
| 30 | | |

## B. Mydriatic and miotic effect on rabbit eye:

### Requirement:

**Animal:** Rabbits (1.5-2.5 kg)

**Drugs:** Ephedrine (4% w/v) and pilocarpine (1% w/v)

**Equipment:** Rabbit holder, dropper, cotton swab, pupilometer.

### Procedure:

1. Place the rabbit in the rabbit holder by keeping the head outside the holder. Acclimatize the rabbit for 5 minute in rabbit holder.
2. Observe the size of the pupil in both the eyes by placing a pupilometer.
3. Prepare stock solution of ephedrine (4% w/v) and pilocarpine (1% w/v).
4. Examine the effect of corneal reflex, light reflex and effect of conjunctiva before and after administration of drugs into the eye.
5. Instill few drops of either ephedrine or pilocarpine solution using dropper in right eye of the rabbit.
6. The left eye would serve as control and instill few drops of normal saline.
7. Record the papillary size, corneal reflex, light reflex and effect of conjunctiva after 5, 10, 20, 30, 60 minute of drug instillation.
8. Compare the response of both control and test eye.

## Observation table:

| Treatment | Time (Min.) | Pupillary Size (mm) | | Corneal Reflex (Present/ Absent) | | Light Reflex (Present/ Absent) | | Effect on conjunctiva | |
|---|---|---|---|---|---|---|---|---|---|
| | | Right Eye | Left Eye | Right Eye | Left Eye | Right Eye | Left Eye | Right Eye | Left Eye |
| Ephedrine | 5 | | | | | | | | |
| | 10 | | | | | | | | |
| | 20 | | | | | | | | |
| | 30 | | | | | | | | |
| | 60 | | | | | | | | |
| Pilocarpine | 5 | | | | | | | | |
| | 10 | | | | | | | | |
| | 20 | | | | | | | | |
| | 30 | | | | | | | | |
| | 60 | | | | | | | | |

## Precautions:

1. Handle the animals with care.
2. Maintain the laboratory conditions properly.

# VIVA-VOCE

**Q.1 Define Mydriatics**

**Ans:** Mydriatics are the drugs that dilate the pupils.

**Q.2 Define Miotics.**

**Ans:** Miotics are the drug which constrict the pupil.

# Experiment No. 10

## Object: To study the effects of skeletal muscle relaxants using rota-rod apparatus.

## Principle:

The loss of muscle grip along with the disturbance in the maintenance of posture and tone is an indication of centrally mediated skeletal muscle relaxant. One of the important pharmacological actions of anti-anxiety agents of benzodiazepine class of drugs is muscle relaxing property. Diazepam causes neurological deficit and cause motor in co-ordination. An untreated mouse trained to remain on the rod at a speed 20 revolution/min for 5 minute, if they fall down earlier when treated with diazepam. The difference in the fall off time from the rotating rod between the control and diazepam treated animal is taken as a index of muscle relaxation. The rod is divided into 2-5 sections for studying the muscle gripping activity in more number of animals at a time. Timer is placed in each section at the base of the instrument. The normal mouse can stay on the rod for a time period 2-3 min. This effect is suggestive of neurological deficit induced by diazepam.

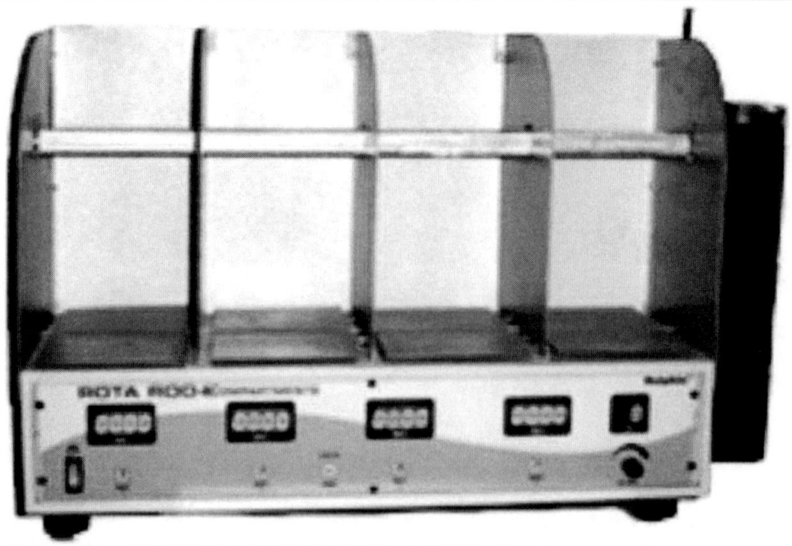

**Rota-rod Apparatus**

## Requirement:

**Animal:** Mice (20-25gm)

**Drugs:** Diazepam (4 mg/kg, i.p)

**Equipment:** Rota rod apparatus

## Procedure:

1. Weigh the animals and randomly divide into two groups i.e. control and test group and each group consist of 6 animals.
2. Turn on the instrument, select an appropriate speed (20-25rpm)
3. Start the rota-rod and place the animal one by one on the rotating rod. One can place more than one mouse.
4. Note down the fall off time when the mouse falls from the rotating rod. A normal mouse generally falls off within 3-5 min
5. Administer saline to control group and diazepam (4 mg/kg, i.p.) to test group mice.
6. After 30 min of drug treatment, again follow the step 3 and note the fall off time.
7. Compare the fall off time of animals before and after diazepam treatment.

## Observation table:

| Group | Body weight (gm) | Drug treatment Dose | Volume of drug injected (ml) | Fall of time (in sec) | | % decrease in activity |
|---|---|---|---|---|---|---|
| | | | | Before drug | After drug | |
| Control | | Saline | | | | |
| | | | | | | |
| | | | | | | |
| | | | | | | |
| | | | | | | |
| | | | | | | |
| Test | | Diazepam 4mg/kg (i.p) | | | | |
| | | | | | | |
| | | | | | | |
| | | | | | | |
| | | | | | | |
| | | | | | | |

## Precautions:

1. Handle the animals with care.
2. Maintain the laboratory conditions properly.
3. Place the animal on the apparatus carefully.

## VIVA-VOCE

**Q.1 Give the principle of rota-rod apparatus.**

**Ans:** An untreated mouse trained to remain on the rod at a speed 20 revolution/min for 5 minute, if they fall down earlier when treated with diazepam. The difference in the fall off time from the rotating rod between the control and diazepam treated animal is taken as a index of muscle relaxation. The rod is divided into 2-5 sections for studying the muscle gripping activity in more number of animals at a time. Timer is placed in each section at the base of the instrument. The normal mouse can stay on the rod for a time period 2-3 min. This effect is suggestive of neurological deficit induced by diazepam.

**Q.2 Explain muscle relaxant activity.**

**Ans:** A muscle relaxant is a drug that affects skeletal muscle function and decreases the muscle tone.

**Q.3 What are the mechanisms of muscle relaxants.**

**Ans:** Muscle relaxants block transmission through the neuromuscular junction (NMJ) at nicotinic receptors, thus decreasing skeletal muscle tone.

# Experiment No. 11

## Object: To study the effect of drugs on locomotor activity using actophotometer.

## Principle:

Most of the central nervous system acting drugs influence the locomotor activities in man and animals. The CNS depressant drugs such as barbiturates and alcohol reduces the motor activity while the stimulants such as caffeine, amphetamines increases the activity.

**CNS Stimulants:** Central nervous system stimulation is the primary action of a various groups of pharmacological agents which selectively enhance the level of activity of specialized cells and hence the adverse effect associated with many drugs.

**CNS Depressants:** CNS depression is the action of different pharmacological agents which causes selective diminution of activity of specialized cells and depresses or slows down the body functions, which can be procured readily from illicit source.

The drugs acting on the central nervous system will affect the motor activities in animals. CNS stimulants increase the locomotor activity while depressants reduce the activity. CNS stimulantion or depression occurs due to imbalance between inhibitory neurotransmitters like GABA, Glycine and excitatory neurotransmitters like glutamate, aspartate in brain system. The locomotor activity can be easily measured using an actophotometer, which operates on photoelectric cells which are connected in circuit with a counter. When the beam of light falling on the photocell is cut off by the animal, a count is recorded. An actophotometer could have either circular or square area in which the animal moves. Both rats and mice may be used for testing in this equipment.

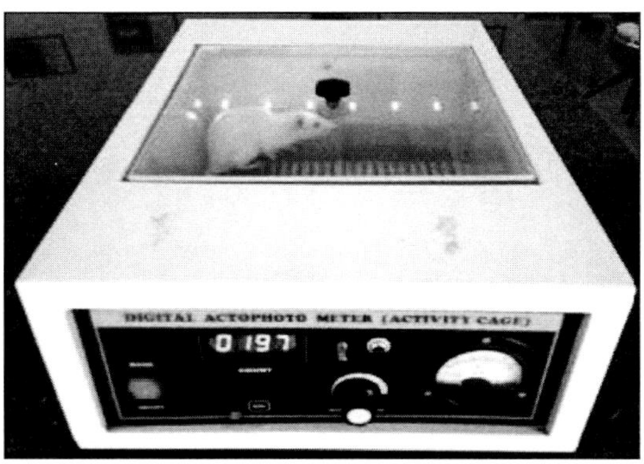


**Actophotometer**

## Requirements:

**Animal:** Mice (20-25gm)

**Drugs:** Chlorpromazine hydrochloride (3 mg/kg)

**Equipment:** Actophotometer

## Procedure:

1. Weigh the animals and number them
2. Turn on the equipment (check and make sure that all the photocells are working for accurate recording) and place individually each mouse in the activity cage for 10 min. Note the basal activity score of all the animals.
3. Inject chlorpromazine (1 ml/100 gm), and after 30 min re –test each mouse for activity scores for 10 min. Note the difference in the activity, before and after chlorpromazine.
4. Calculate percent decrease in motor activity.

## Observation table:

| S.No | Body weight (gm) | Drug treatment dose | Volume of drug injected (ml) | Locomotor Activity (Scores) in 10 min | | % decrease in activity |
|---|---|---|---|---|---|---|
| | | | | Before drug | After drug | |
| 1. | | Chlorpromazine 3mg/kg (i.p) | | | | |
| 2. | | | | | | |
| 3. | | | | | | |
| 4. | | | | | | |
| 5. | | | | | | |
| 6. | | | | | | |
| Mean | | | | | | |

## Precautions:

1. Handle the animals with care.
2. Maintain the laboratory conditions properly.
3. Place the animal on the apparatus carefully.

# VIVA-VOCE

**Q.1 Give the principal of actophotometer.**

**Ans:** The locomotor activity can be easily measured using an actophotometer. Which operates on photoelectric cells which are connected in circuit with a counter. When the beam of light falling on the photocell is cut off by the animal, a count is recorded. An actophotometer could have either circular or square arena in which the animal moves.

**Q.2 Explain the effect of drug on motor activity.**

**Ans:** The drugs which acting on the central nervous system will affect the motor activities in animals. CNS stimulants increase the locomotor activity while depressants reduce the activity. CNS stimulantion or depression occurs due to imbalance between inhibitory neurotransmitters like GABA, Glycine and excitatory neurotransmitters like glutamate, aspartate in brain system.

**Q.3 Define CNS Stimulants.**

**Ans:** Central nervous system stimulation is the primary action of a various groups of pharmacological agents which selectively enhance the level of activity of specialized cells and hence the adverse effect associated with many drugs.

**Q.4 Define CNS Depressants.**

**Ans:** CNS depression is the action of different pharmacological agents which causes selective diminution of activity of specialized cells and depresses or slowing down the body functions, which can be procured readily from illicit source.

# Experiment No. 12

## Object: To study anti-convulsant effect of drugs by MES and PTZ method.

## Principle:

The convulsion in rat and mice can be induced by giving high voltage current near the brain or by suitable CNS stimulants (Eg. Pentylenetetrazol). The screening of antiepileptic agents can be done by experimentally induced convulsion (Seizures) and their prevention by drug under test.

## Maximal electro-shock-induced convulsions:

In MES- convulsions electroshock is applied through the corneal electrodes. Through optic stimulation cortical excitation is produced. The MES convulsions are divided into five phases such as (a) Tonic flexion; (b) Tonic extensor; (c) Clonic convulsion; (d)Stupor (e) Recovery / death.

A substance is known to possess anticonvulsant property if it reduces or abolishes the extensor phase of MES convulsions. This procedure may be used to study convulsions both in rats and mice.

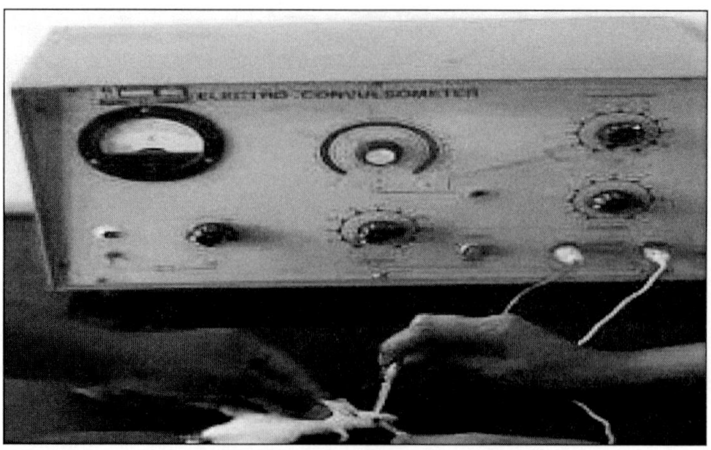

**Electro- convulsiometer**

## Requirement:

**Animal:** Rats (150-200 gm)

**Drugs:** Phenytoin (dose 25 mg/kg)

**Equipment:** Electro- convulsiometer, cornel electrode (150 mA current for 0.2 sec), Stop watch.

## Procedure:

1. Weigh and number the animals.
2. Divide them into two groups each consisting of 4-5 rats.
3. One group is used as control and the other for drugs treatment.
4. Hold the animals properly, place corneal electrodes on the cornea and apply the prescribed current. Note the different stages of convulsions: (a) Tonic flexion; (b) Tonic extensor; (c) Clonic convulsion; (d) Stupor (e) Recovery / death.
5. Note the time (sec) spent by the animal in each phase of the convulsions.
6. Repeat with other animals of control group
7. Inject phenytoin I.P to group of 4-5 rats.
8. Wait for 30 min and subject the animals to electroconvulsions.
9. Note the reduction in time or abolition of tonic extensor phase of MES convulsions.

## Observation table:

| S.No. | Body wt. | Treatment (Dose) | Time (sec) in various phases of convulsion | | | | |
|---|---|---|---|---|---|---|---|
| | | | Flexion | Extensor | Clonus | Stupor | Recovery/Death |
| 1. | | Control (Saline) | | | | | |
| 2. | | | | | | | |
| 3. | | | | | | | |
| 4. | | | | | | | |
| 5. | | | | | | | |
| Mean | | | | | | | |
| 1. | | Phenytoin | | | | | |
| 2. | | | | | | | |
| 3. | | | | | | | |
| 4. | | | | | | | |
| 5. | | | | | | | |
| Mean | | | | | | | |

## Pentylenetetrazol-induced convulsions (PTZ):

Pentylenetetrazol is a central nervous system stimulant. It produces jerky type of clonic convulsions in rat and mice. The convulsive effect of this drug is considered to be analogus to petit mal type of convulsions in man. Recently pentylenetetrazol has been reported to act through GABA-benzodiazepine receptor mechanisms in the brain. It is widely used as a tool in experimental pharmacology to study convulsions and anticonvulsant action of drugs.

### Requirement:

**Animal:** Mice (20-25 gm)

**Drugs:** Pentylenetetrazol (dose 80 mg/kg); Diazepam (dose 4 mg/kg)

### Procedure:

1. Weigh and number the animals.
2. Divide them into two groups each consisting of 5 mice.
3. One group is used for studying the effect of pentylenetetrazol alone (control) and other for studying the protective effect of diazepam.
4. Inject pentylenetetrazol to control animals and note the onset of action (indicated by Straub's tail, jerky movements of whole body and convulsions) and severity of convulsion due to the drug.
5. Inject diazepam to second group. After 30 min inject pentylenetetrazol to these animals which have received diazepam. Note onset and severity of convulsions.
6. Note either delay or complete abolition of convulsions in mice treated with diazepam.

### Observation table:

| S.No. | Body wt. | Treatment (Dose) | Convulsions Time in (sec) | | | | |
|---|---|---|---|---|---|---|---|
| | | | Onset of jerks | Onset of clonus | Duration of clonus | Onset of extensor | Recovery/ Death |
| 1. | | PTZ | | | | | |
| 2. | | | | | | | |
| 3. | | | | | | | |
| 4. | | | | | | | |
| 5. | | | | | | | |
| Mean | | | | | | | |

| S.No. | Body wt. | Treatment (Dose) | Convulsions Time in (sec) | | | | |
|---|---|---|---|---|---|---|---|
| | | | Onset of jerks | Onset of clonus | Duration of clonus | Onset of extensor | Recovery/ Death |
| 1. | | Diazepam + PTZ | | | | | |
| 2. | | | | | | | |
| 3. | | | | | | | |
| 4. | | | | | | | |
| 5. | | | | | | | |
| Mean | | | | | | | |

## Precautions:

1. Handle the animals with care.
2. Maintain the laboratory conditions properly.
3. Place the animal on the apparatus carefully.

# VIVA-VOCE

**Q.1 Give the principle of anti-convulsant activity using convulsiometer.**

**Ans:** The convulsion in rat and mice can be induced by giving high voltage current near the brain or by suitable CNS stimulants (Eg. Pentylenetetrazol). The screening of antiepileptic agents can be done by experimentally induced convulsion (Seizures) and their prevention by drug under test.

**Q.2 Explain Pentylenetetrazol-induced convulsions (PTZ).**

**Ans:** Pentylenetetrazol is a central nervous system stimulant. It produces jerky type of clonic convulsions in rat and mice. The convulsive effect of this drug is considered to be analogus to petit mal type of convulsions in man. Recently pentylenetetrazol has been reported to act through GABA-benzodiazepine receptor mechanisms in the brain. It is widely used as a tool in experimental pharmacology to study convulsions and anticonvulsant action of drugs.

**Q.3 Explain Maximal electro-shock-induced convulsions.**

**Ans:** In MES- convulsions electroshock is applied through the corneal electrodes. Through optic stimulation cortical excitation is produced. The MES convulsions are divided into five phases such as (a) Tonic flexion; (b) Tonic extensor; (c) Clonic convulsion; (d) Stupor

(e) Recovery / death. A substance is known to possess anticonvulsant property if it reduces or abolishes the extensor phase of MES convulsions. This procedure may be used to study convulsions both in rats and mice.

**Q.4 Explain phases of Maximal electro-shock-induced convulsions.**

**Ans:** The MES convulsions are divided into five phases such as (a) Tonic flexion; (b) Tonic extensor; (c) Clonic convulsion; (d) Stupor (e) Recovery / death.

# Experiment No. 13

## Object: To study the stereotype and anti-catatonic activity of drugs on rats/mice.

### Principle:

Phenothiazine and butyrophenone type of antipsychotic drugs are known to produce extrapyramidal side-effects in man. These effects, such as akinesia, rigidity and tremors, are called parkinson's- like because in parkinson's disease the major clinical symptoms include difficulty to move and change posture (akinesia and rigidity) and tremors. These effects of antipsychotic drugs are due to excessive blockade of dopamine receptors in the extrapyramidal motor system. Therefore, phenothiazines (choloropromazine or perphenazine) are commonly used to produce parkinson's-like extrapyramidal symptoms in laboratory animals and to study anti-parkinsonism drugs. The students are advised to know the pharmacology of anti-parkinsonism drugs before performing this experiment.

### Requirements:

**Animal:** Rats (150-200 g)

**Drugs:** Perphenazine (5 mg/kg i.p.), Scopolamine (2 mg/kg, i.p.)

**Equipment:** Two wooden blocks, one being 3 cm high and the other 9 cm high

### Procedure:

1. Weigh and number the animal. Divide the animals into two groups, one for control (for study of perphenazine effect) and the other for studying the effects of scopolamine. Each group should consist of at least 5 animals.
2. Inject perphenazine to control animals. observe severity of catatonic response as follows:

| Stages | Description | Score |
|---|---|---|
| Stage – I | Rat moves normally when placed on table | 0 |
| Stage – II | Rat moves only when touched or pushed | 0.5 |
| Stage – III | Rat placed on the table with front paws set alternatively on a 3 cm high block fail to correct the posture in 10 seconds | 0.5 (for each paw With a total score 1) |

| Stages | Description | Score |
|---|---|---|
| Stage – IV | Rat placed on the table with front paws set alternatively on a 9 cm long block fail to correct the posture in 10 seconds | 1 (for each paw with a total score 2) |

Thus for a single rat, the maximum possible score would be (0.5+1+2) 3.5 revealing total catatonia.

3. Observe the severity of catatonia at 5, 15, 30, 45, 60, 90 and 120 min after perphenazine.
4. To the second group inject scopolamine and after 30 minute inject perphenazine to these animals already treated with scopolamine. Observe and score the severity of catatonic as in step 2.
5. Compare the onset and severity of catatonic response in the both groups. Plot a graph, time along the x-axis. Note the difference in the onset and severity of catatonic response in both the groups.

## Observation table:

| S.No. | Body wt. (gm) | Treatment (mg/kg) | Degree of catatonic response after min. | | | | | | |
|---|---|---|---|---|---|---|---|---|---|
| | | | 5 | 15 | 30 | 45 | 60 | 90 | 120 |
| 1. | | Perphenazine | | | | | | | |
| 2. | | | | | | | | | |
| 3. | | | | | | | | | |
| 4. | | | | | | | | | |
| 5. | | | | | | | | | |
| Mean | | | | | | | | | |
| 1. | | Scopolamine + Perphenazine | | | | | | | |
| 2. | | | | | | | | | |
| 3. | | | | | | | | | |
| 4. | | | | | | | | | |
| 5. | | | | | | | | | |
| Mean | | | | | | | | | |

## Precautions:

1. Handle the animals with care.
2. Maintain the laboratory conditions properly.

## VIVA-VOCE

**Q.1 Define catatonia.**

**Ans:** Catatonia is a complex neuropsychiatric behavioral syndrome that is characterized by abnormal movements, immobility, abnormal behaviors and withdrawal.

**Q.2 Define parkinsonism.**

**Ans:** Parkinsonism is a clinical syndrome characterized by tremor, bradykinesia (slowed movements), rigidity and postural instability

# Experiment No. 14

## Object: To study the anxiolytic activity of drugs using rats/mice.

## Introduction:

- Anxiety is chronic condition characterized by an excessive and persistent sense of apprehension with physical symptoms such as sweating, palpitations, and feelings of stress. Anxiety disorders have biological and environmental causes.
- Anxiety is a commonly experienced emotion. It is an uncomfortable feeling of apprehension or fear coupled with sensations of physical arousal.
- If anxiety is excessive or interferes with functioning, it is considered a pathologic anxiety disorder.
- Anxiety is different from fear due to its cognitive component (i.e. fear of the future)
- Anxiety can be helpful and adaptive (e.g. anxiety about giving lectures!)
- An anxiety disorder may be a primary disorder or it may occur secondary to medical causes or substances (e.g., medications or illicit substances); it may occur as a response to acute stressors or it may be associated with another psychiatric disorder.

## Types of Anxiety Disorders:

1) Generalized Anxiety Disorder
2) Panic Disorder
3) Phobic Disorders - Agoraphobia, Acrophobia,Aquaphobia
4) Obsessive-Compulsive Disorder
5) Post-Traumatic Stress Disorder

## MODELS FOR ANTIANXIETY ACTIVITY FOR RATS/MICE:

### 1. Elevated plus maze test:

#### Principle:

There are various number of models in use for studying the anxiolytic activity in animals. Elevated plus-maze is the simplest apparatus to study anxiety response and the effect of almost all type of anti-anxiety agents. It is more simple apparatus, reliable, less time consuming and can study the effect of almost all types of anti-anxiety agents. The plus-maze apparatus consists of two open arms (16x5 cm for mouse and 50x10 cm for rats; LxW) and two enclosed arms (16x5x12 cm for mouse and 50x10x40 cm for rats; LxWxH), open to top, arranged so that two open arms are opposite to each other. The maze is elevated at height of 25 cm for mice and 50 cm for rats from the floor. Rats and mice prefer enclosed arm than open and high space. So, when animals enter into open, they freeze, become immobile, defecate and show fear like movements. The plasma cortisol level is also reported to be increased, as a true event of anxiety. Motor activity and open arm exploratory time are registered. Benzodiazepine decrease motor activity and increase open arm exploratory time. The animals are placed individually in the center of the maze, with their head facing towards open arm. The observation during 5 minute of time interval is:

- Preference of first entry of animal
- Number of entries in open arm and closed arm
- Time spent in open and close arm

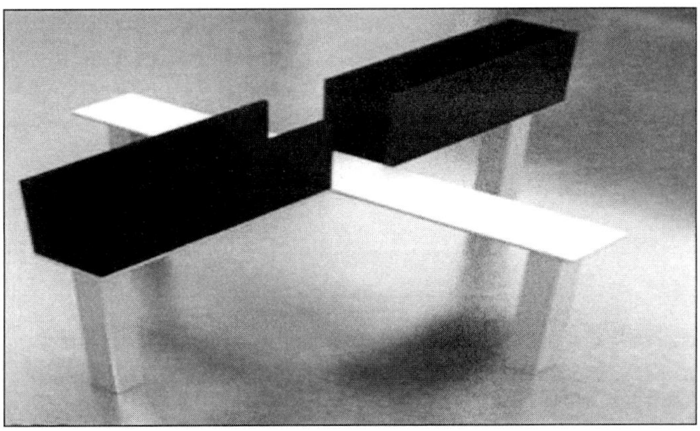

**Elevated plus maze apparatus**

## Requirements:

**Animal:** Wistar albino rat (180-200)

**Drugs:** Diazepam (1.0 mg/ml), Saline

**Equipments:** Elevated plus maze apparatus, stop watch, syringes and needle.

## Purpose and Rationale:

- Out of many possibilities to modify maze tests e.g. water maze, the Y-mace, the radial maze and the elevated plus maze have found acceptance in many laboratories.
- The test has been proposed for selective identification of anxiolytic and anxiogenic drugs.
- Anxiolytic compounds, by decreasing anxiety, increase the open arm exploration time; anxiogenic compounds have the opposite effect.

## Procedure:

1. The plus-maze consists of two open arms, 50 × 10 × 40 cm, and two enclosed arms, 50 × 10 × 40 cm, with an open roof, arranged such that the two open arms are opposite to each other.
2. The maze is elevated to a height of 50 cm. The rats (200–250 g body weight) are housed in pairs for 10 days prior to testing in the apparatus.
3. During this time the rats are handled by the investigator on alternate days to reduce stress.
4. Groups consist of 6 rats for each dose.
5. Thirty min after i.p. administration of the test drug or the standard, the rat is placed in the center of the maze, facing one of the enclosed arms.
6. During a 5 min test period the following measures are taken:
7. The number of entries into and time spent in the open and enclosed arms.
8. The total number of arm entries.

## Observation table:

| Group | S.No. | Weight | First preference arm of the rats | | Total number of entries | | Time spent in the arms (Sec.) | |
|---|---|---|---|---|---|---|---|---|
| Control (Saline) | 1 | | | | | | | |
| | 2 | | | | | | | |
| | 3 | | | | | | | |
| | 4 | | | | | | | |
| | 5 | | | | | | | |
| | 6 | | | | | | | |
| | Mean | | | | | | | |
| Test (Diazepam) | 1 | | | | | | | |
| | 2 | | | | | | | |
| | 3 | | | | | | | |
| | 4 | | | | | | | |
| | 5 | | | | | | | |
| | 6 | | | | | | | |
| | Mean | | | | | | | |

### Evaluation:

Motor activity and open arm exploratory time are registered. The values of treated groups are expressed as percentage of controls. Benzodiazepines and valproate decrease motor activity and increase open arm exploratory time.

### Precautions:

1. Handle the animals with care.
2. Acclimatize the animals prior to testing in the apparatus.
3. Maintain the laboratory conditions properly.

## 2. Anti-anxiety test (Light-dark model):

### Purpose and Rationale:

- Crawley and Goodwin (1980) Crawley (1981) described a simple behavior model in mice to detect compounds with anxiolytic effects. Mice and rats tend to explore a novel environment.
- In a two chambered system, where the animals can freely move between a brightly open field and a dark corner.
- They show more crossings between the two chambers and more locomotor activity after treatment with anxiolytics.
- The number of crossings between the light and dark sites are recorded.

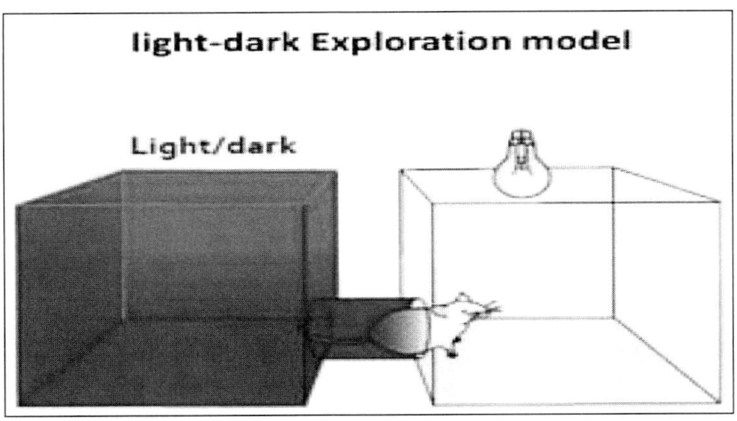


### Procedure:

1. The testing apparatus consists of a light and a dark chamber divided by a photocell-equipped zone.

2. A animal cage, 44 × 21 × 21 cm, is darkened with black spray over one-third of its surface.
3. A partition containing a 13 cm long × 5 cm high opening separates the dark one third from the bright two thirds of the cage.
4. An electronic system using four sets of photocells across the partition automatically counts movements through the partition and clocks the time spent in the light and dark compartments.
5. Male mice or rats are placed into the cage.
6. The animals are treated 30 min before the experiment with the test drugs or the vehicle intraperitoneally and are then observed for 10 min.
7. Groups of 6–8 animals are used for each dose.

### Evaluation:

Dose-response curves are obtained and the number of crossings through the partition between the light and the dark chamber are compared with total activity counts during the 10 min.

## 3. Anticipatory anxiety in mice:

### Purpose and Rationale:

- When group-housed mice are removed one by one from their home cage, the last mice removed have always higher rectal temperatures than those removed first .
- This phenomenon is interpreted as being caused by anticipatory fear for an aversive event.
- This test is thought to be a model of anticipatory anxiety.

### Procedure:

1. Groups of 18 male albino Swiss mice weighing 25–30 gm are used.
2. Test drugs or standard (diazepam) or solvent are administered orally in various doses to groups of 18 mice prior to the test.
3. Thirty min later, the first 3 mice are removed from the cage and the rectal temperature measured by inserting a silicone lubricated thermistor probe (2 mm diameter) for 2.5 cm into the rectum.
4. The average temperature of these 3 mice is taken as basal value.
5. Thereafter body temperature is determined in the remaining three animals.
6. The difference of the mean value of these mice and the basal values is calculated as increase. Vehicle treated test groups display increase of 1.1 to 1.3 °C.

## Evaluation:

The mean increase values of treated groups ±SEM are compared by ANOVA statistics with the controls.

## 4. Social interaction in rats:

### Purpose and Rationale:

- In an unfamiliar and brightly lit environment, the normal social interaction of rats (e.g. sniffing, nipping, grooming) is suppressed.
- Anxiolytics counteract this suppression.

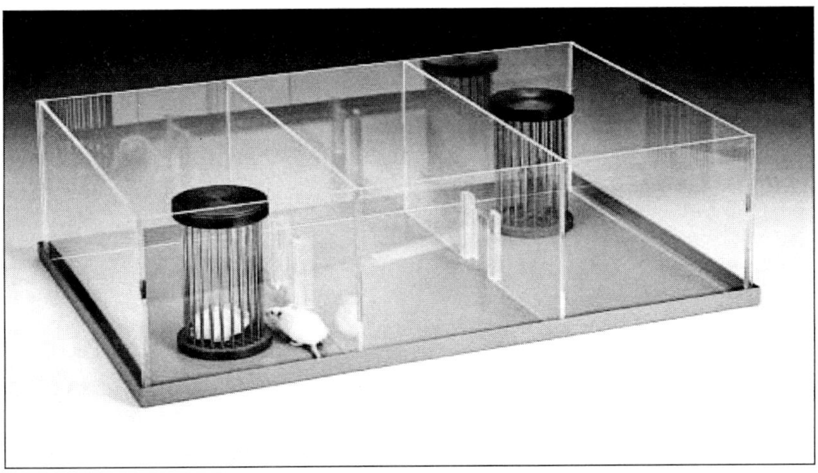

**Social interaction model**

### Procedure:

1. Male Sprague-Dawley rats (225–275 gm body weight) are housed in groups of 5 animals.
2. The apparatus used for the detection of changes in social behavior and exploratory behavior consists of a open-topped box (51 × 51 cm and 20 cm high) with 17 × 17 cm marked areas on the floor.
3. One hour prior to the test, two naive rats from separate housing cages are treated with the test compound orally. They are placed in to the box and their behavior is observed over a 10-min period by remote video recording.
4. Two types of behavior can be noted:
   - ➢ Social interaction between the animals is determined by timing the sniffing of partner, crawling under or climbing over the partner, genital investigation of partner.

- ➢ Exploratory motion is measured as the number of crossings of the lines marked on the floor of the test box.
- ➢ Six pairs are used for each dose.

## Evaluation:

The values of treated partners are compared with the data from 6 pairs of untreated animals using single factor analysis of variance followed by Dunnett's-test.

## 5. Water maze test:

### Purpose and Rationale:

Spatial learning of rats can be tested in a water maze

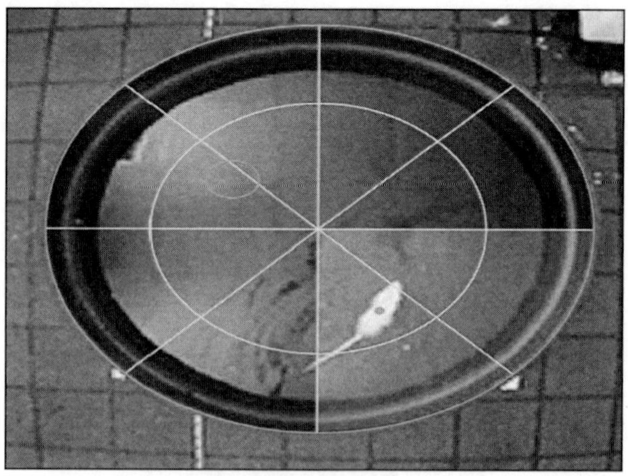

**Water maze test**

### Procedure:

1. The water maze consists of a circular tank with 100 cm diameter and a wall 20 cm above the water level.
2. A circular platform (9 cm diameter) is hidden 2 cm below the water level.
3. The water is made opaque using titanium dioxide suspension and is kept at about 23 °C during the experiment.
4. Training takes place on three consecutive days, with the rats receiving 4 consecutive trials per day with an trial interval of 6–10 min.
5. Latency to find the platform is measured as the time of placement of the rat in the water to the time it finds the platform.
6. If the animal fails to find the platform in any trial within 3 min it is placed on it for 10 s.

### Evaluation:

- The platform is removed and the time spent in the target quadrant (the quadrant in the center of which the platform has been located) and the number of annulus crossings across the actual location where the platform has been located in the first 60 s of exposure are measured.
- The time to the first annulus crossing is taken as a measure of performance of trial.
- Buspirone as well as benzodiazepines increase the latency to find the platform in the training period and impair the number and the time of annulus crossings.

## 7. Staircase test:

### Purpose and Rationale:

- When introduced into a novel environment, rodents experience a conflict between anxiety and exploratory behavior manifested by increased vigilance and behavioral activity.
- In the staircase paradigm, step-climbing is purported to reflect exploratory or locomotor activity, while rearing behavior is an index of anxiety state.
- The number of rearings and steps climbed are recorded in a 5 min period.
- The dissociation of these parameters is considered to be characteristic for anxiolytic drugs.

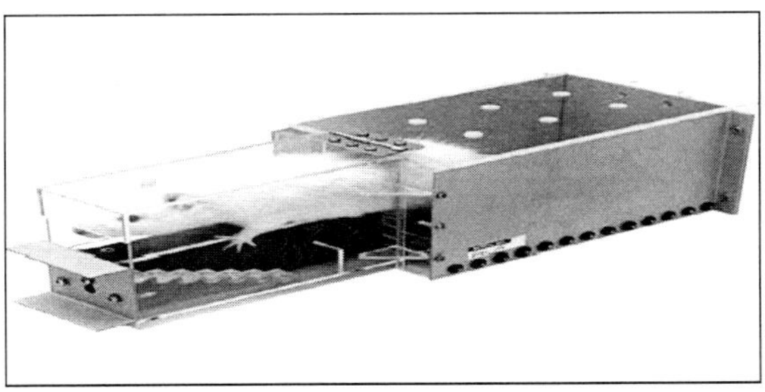

**Staircase**

### Procedure:

1. For experiments with mice the staircase is composed of five identical steps 2.5 cm high, 10 cm wide and 7.5 cm deep.
2. Male mice with a weight between 18 and 24 g are used. Each animal is used only once.
3. The drug or the standard is administered orally 1 h or 30 min subcutaneously before the test. The animal is placed on the floor of the box with its back to the staircase.
4. The number of steps climbed and the number of rears are counted over a 3-min period.

### Evaluation:

- Twelve mice are used for the untreated control group and for the group receiving the standard.
- The average number of steps and rearings of the control group is taken as 100%.
- The values of treated animals are expressed as percentage of the controls.

## 7. Cork gnawing test in the rat:

### Purpose and Rationale:

1. Cork gnawing behavior in the rat has been proposed as a screening method for buspirone- like anxiolytics.

### Procedure:

1. Adult male evans rats serve as subjects.
2. They are housed 4 per cage on a regular light/dark cycle with free access to food and water
3. For the test session one animal is placed in a stainless steel cage with wire mesh bottom.
4. A session consists of placing the subject in the test cage with a cork stopper weighing between 2–3 gm for 30 min.
5. Initially, the amount gnawed is relatively high and variable within and between subjects. After 30 training sessions, the amount is low and stabilized.
6. The test compounds are injected 30 min before the test and food is withdrawn.
7. The average cork loss during the previous control days is taken as baseline and the amount after drug treatment is expressed as percentage of baseline.
8. Buspirone-related compounds as well as benzodiazepines and meprobamate show a dose dependent increase of cork gnawing.

### Evaluation:

- Each cork is weighed to the nearest 0.01 g before and after the session

## 8. Schedule induced polydipsia in rats:

### Purpose and Rationale:

- Food deprived rats exposed to a procedure in which food is delivered intermittently will drink large amounts of water if given the opportunity to do so.
- This behavioral phenomenon is termed schedule-induced.

## Procedure:

- Male wistar rats weighing 180–250 g are individually housed at a 12 h/12 h light/dark cycle for a 1 week acclimation period with free access to food and water.
- Then they are placed on a restricted diet which maintains 80% of their free feeding body weight.
- To induce polydipsia, rats are placed in test chambers housed in sound attenuated boxes where a pellet dispenser automatically dispenses two 45 mg pellets on a fixed time 60-s feeding schedule over a 150 min test session.
- Water is available at all times in the test chambers.
- After 4 weeks exposure to the 60s feeding schedule, approximately 80% of the rats meet the pre-determined criterion for water consumption (greater than 60 ml water per session) and are considered to have polydipsic behavior.

## Evaluation:

The experimental data comparing the effects of chronic administration of compounds on schedule-induced polydipsia are analyzed with the Mann Whitney U-test.

## 9. Four plate test in mice:

### Purpose and Rationale

The four plate test in mice has been used for the rapid screening of minor tranquilizers.

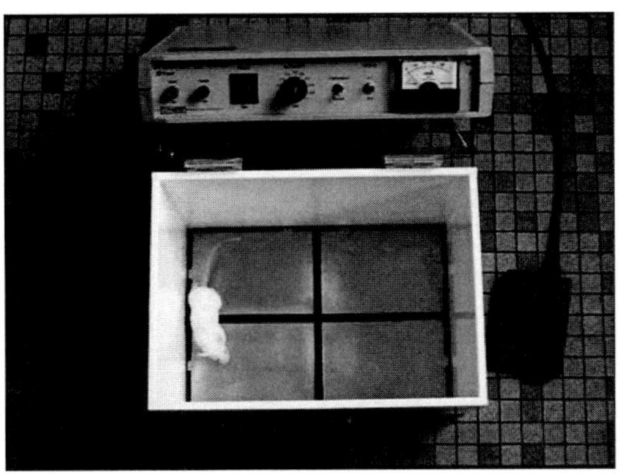

**Four plate**

## Procedure:

1. The test box has the shape of a rectangle (25 × 18 × 16 cm).
2. The floor is covered with 4 identical rectangular metal plates (8 × 11 cm) separated from one another by a gap of 4 mm.

3. The plates are connected to a source of continuous current which applies to 2 adjacent plates a mild electrical shock of 0.35 mA for 0.5 s. This evokes a clear flight reaction of the animals.
4. Adult male Swiss albino mice, weighing 17 to 23 g, are randomly divided into different groups.
5. Thirty min before the test the animals are injected intraperitoneally with the test drug or the vehicle.
6. At the beginning of the test, the mouse is gently dropped on to a plate and is allowed to explore the enclosure for 15 s.
7. After this, every time the animal crosses from one plate to another, the experimenter electrifies the whole floor for 0.5 s, which evokes a clear flight-reaction of the mouse.

### Evaluation:

- The number of times the apparatus is electrified is counted each minute for 10 min.
- The delivery of shocks decreases dramatically the motor activity.
- The number of shocks received during the first min is taken as parameter. This number is increased by minor tranquilizers, such as benzodiazepines.

## 10. Foot shock induced freezing behavior in rats:

### Purpose and Rationale:

Foot shock-induced freezing behavior in rats has been proposed as a model for anxiolytics.

### Procedure:

1. Male Sprague-Dawley rats with a weight between 200 and 350 g are used.
2. The animals receive a single i.p. injection of the test compound or the vehicle 30 min prior to being placed in a standard conditioning chamber (e.g. Coulborn Instruments) for a 6.5 min session.
3. 2 and 2.5 min after the start of the session, a foot shock (0.5 mA, 0.5 s) is delivered through the grid floor of the chamber. Following exclusive behaviors are observed:
   - Freezing: immobility with rigid body posture
   - Sedated posture: sitting or sleeping
   - Small exploratory movements: movements involving the torso or front paws only, vertical movements of the head, or sniffing.
   - Locomotion: activity involving hind paws, grooming or rearing. Frequency of rearing is also counted. All behaviors are monitored for the entire 6.5 min session.

### Evaluation:

- Duration of foot-shock induced freezing after the second shock is taken as the critical parameter.
- Time spent in freezing posture after administration of test compounds is compared with the controls.

## 11. mCPP induced anxiety in rats:

### Purpose and Rationale:

- The metabolite of the antidepressant drug trazodone 1- (3-chlorphenyl) piperazine (=mCPP), classified as 5- HT1C agonist or 5-HT1B/2C agonist has been shown to be anxiogenic.
- Antagonism against these symptoms has been proposed as a screening model for anxiolytic drugs.

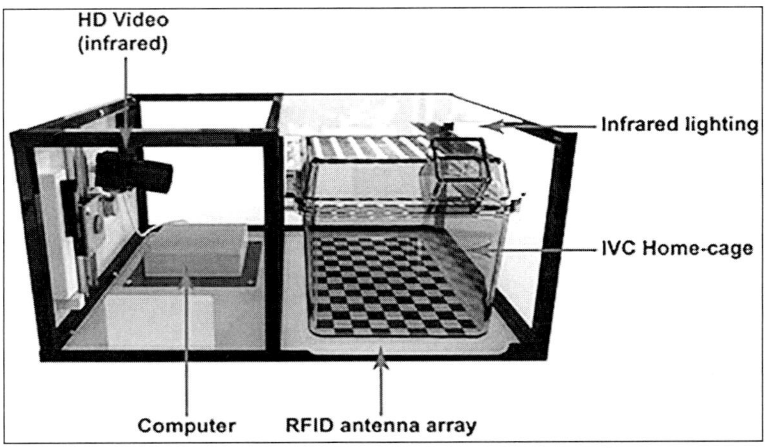


**Automated locomotor activity cages**

### Procedure:

- Male Sprague Dawley rats (220–250 g) are housed in groups of 6 under a 12 h light/dark cycle with free access to food and water.

### mCPP - induced locomotion:

- Rats are used.
- They are dosed either orally 1 h, or i.p. 30 min before the locomotion test with test compound or vehicle, and injected 20 min before the test with 7 mg/kg mCPP i.p. or saline in groups of four.

- At 0 h they are each placed in automated locomotor activity cages.
- locomotion is recorded by means of alternately breaking two photocell beams traversing opposite ends of the box 3.9 cm above floor level.

### mCPP-induced hypophagia:

- Rats are individually housed on day 1 and on day 3 they are deprived of food.
- Twenty-three hours later, they are orally treated with the test drug or vehicle.
- Forty min later, they are given 5 mg/kg mCPP or saline i.p.
- After a further 20 min, weighted amounts of their normal food pellets are placed in their food hoppers and the amount remaining after 1 h is measured.

### Evaluation:

- The effect of the test compound on mCPP-induced hypolocomotion is determined by one-way ANOVA and Newman-Keuls test. The dose producing 50% disinhibition of mCPP is also estimated.
- Feeding test data are subjected to one-way ANOVA and Dunnett's test.

## 12. Acoustic startle response in rats:

### Purpose and Rationale:

- The acoustic startle reflex is a relatively simple behavior that occurs naturally in mammals.
- It consists of a series of rapid movements beginning at the head and contraction and extension of major muscle groups.
- Startle response can be used to determine sites and mechanisms of drug action

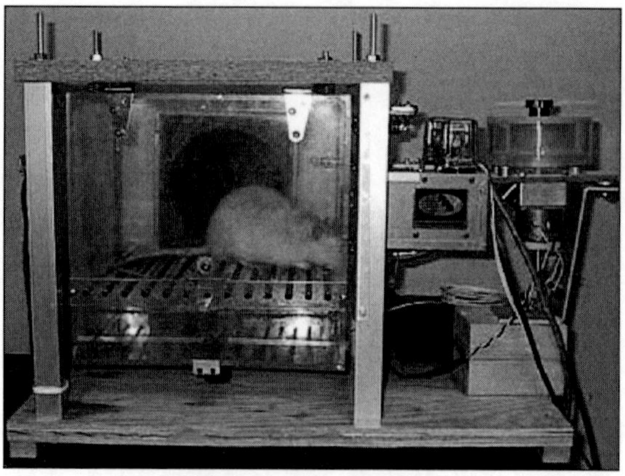

**Acoustic startle**

### Procedure:

1. Male Wistar rats weighing about 200 g are used.
2. Acoustic startle reflexes are measured in a specially build apparatus, e.g., Coulborn Instruments Acoustic Response Test System.
3. The animals are individually placed in 8 × 8 × 16 cm open air cages that restrict locomotion but do not immobilize the animal.
4. Sound-attenuating acoustic chamber is used, when sound is produced physical movement is measured.
5. Data are recorded automatically by an interfaced microcomputer. Pre-tests are performed with all animals to obtain control values.
6. The animals are treated 2 h prior the experiment with test drugs or vehicle given orally or subcutaneously.

### Evaluation:

- The results are given as percentage of the change, related to the values obtained in the pre- test and assessed by a one-way ANOVA, followed by Dunnett's test when appropriate.

## 13. Unconditioned conflict procedure (Vogel test):

### Purpose and Rationale:

- Described a simple and reliable conflict procedure for testing anti-anxiety agents.
- Thirsty, naive rats were administered shocks while licking water.

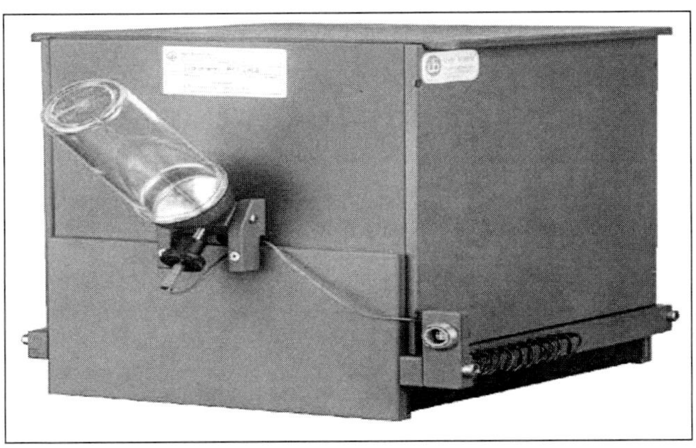

**Lickometer**

### Procedure:

1. The apparatus is a clear Plexiglas box (black in color), The entire apparatus has a stainless- steel grid floor.
2. A water bottle with a metal drinking tube is fitted to the outside of the small compartment, so that the tube is extended into the box at a height 3 cm above the grid.
3. Rats lick at constant rate of 7 licks per sec. A drinkometer circuit is connected between the drinking tube and the grid floor of the apparatus, so that the rat completes the circuit whenever it licks the tube.
4. Shock is administered to the feet of the animal.
5. Thirty min after i.p injection, the rat is placed in the apparatus and allowed to find the drinking tube and to complete 20 licks before shock is administered.
6. The rat controls shock duration by withdrawing from the tube.
7. A 3-min timer is automatically started after the termination of the first shock. During the 3-min period, shocks are delivered following each twentieth lick.
8. The number of shocks delivered during the 3-min session is recorded for each animal.

### Evaluation:

- The number of shocks received after treatment is compared with untreated animals. Benzodiazepines increase dose-dependent number of shocks. Barbiturates at low doses are active in this test.

## 14. Novelty-suppressed feeding:

### Purpose and Rationale:

- Placing a hungry rat into an unfamiliar environment with access to food results in a suppression of feeding behavior relative to the condition when the test environment is familiar.
- This effect has been termed hyponeophagia and occurs because of the novelty of the test environment. The avoidance of novel foods is termed food neophobia.
- Both hyponeophagia and food neophobia have been assumed to measure anxiety by eliciting a conflict situation arising from a fear of the novel setting and foods, and the drive to eat.

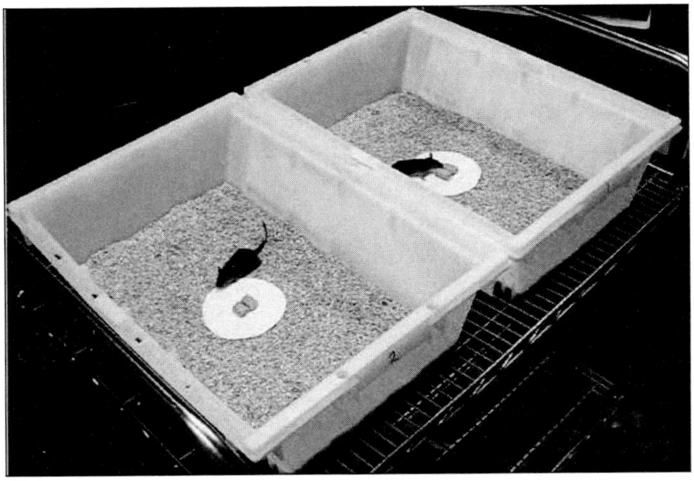

**Novelty-Suppressed feeding**

### Procedure:

1. The testing apparatus consists of individual Plexiglas open fields, 76 × 76 × 46 cm.
2. Thirty Purina lab chow pellets are placed in a pile directly in the center of the open field. Animals are handled for 3 weeks prior the behavioral testing.
3. Forty-eight hours prior to testing, all food is removed from the home cage, although water is still available. One h prior to testing, animals receive an intraperitoneal injection of test drugs or vehicle.
4. At the time of testing, the animals are placed into individual open fields containing the food, and the latency to begin eating is measured.
5. If the animal has not eaten within 720 s, the test is terminated and the animal is assigned a latency score of 720 s.

### Evaluation:

- An anxiolytic effect is defined as a significant decrease in mean latency to begin eating compared with vehicle controls.

## 15. Shock probe conflict procedure:

### Purpose and Rationale:

- Rats being placed in a novel test environment containing a probe.
- Number of times that the animal makes physical contact with it, is reduced when the probe is electrified.
- Rats treated with anxiolytics continue to touch the electrified probe.

### Procedure:

1. Apparatus: The test environment consists of a Plexiglas chamber, measuring 40 × 40 × 40 cm, and having a metal grid floor.
2. Whenever the animal touches both wires simultaneously with some part of its body, a DC current flows through the animal.
3. Sixty min after treatment with saline or test substance, the animal is placed in a back corner of the test box facing away from the probe.
4. The number of responses the animal makes during the subsequent 5-min episode is counted.

### Evaluation:

- Dose-response curves can be established for various drugs at different shock intensities.
- The Mann-Whitney U-test is used to evaluate differences between experimental conditions.
- To control whether a drug treatment increases responding above the saline control level, and one-tail test is used.

## 16. Ultrasound induced defensive behavior in rats:

### Purpose and Rationale:

- Production of ultra-sonic cells in the range of 20–27 kHz are used,
- Rats display specific defence behavior as a part of their natural survival strategy.

### Procedure:

1. The apparatus consists of a circular open field 75 cm in diameter, 46 cm high walls, with a video camera suspended above.
2. Locomotor behaviors are recorded and analyzed using a computer automated tracking system capable of rapid movements. This allows the ultrasound induced change in locomotor behavior to be quantified in maximum speed, average speed and distance travelled by the animals.
3. Animals are placed in the test arena 20 min after intraperitoneal injection of drug or vehicle and locomotor activity is measured.
4. After 2 min they are exposed to a 1-min, 20 kHz, square wave ultrasound tone followed by a further 2 min without sound. This procedure is repeated for each intensity with a 1- min interval.
5. Locomotor activity values are then calculated for the maximum speed, average speed and total distance travelled throughout the 5-min test period is expressed as a series of 15–20s.

### Evaluation:

- Maximum speed is analyzed using a two-way ANOVA.
- Significant interactions between treatment and time are followed by one-way ANOVAs for individual time points with post-hoc Duncan's new multiple range test.

## 17. Anxiety/Defense test battery in rats:

### Purpose and Rationale

- It is the procedure designed to assess the defensive reactions of rats to a natural predator, the cat.
- The primary measures, taken both during and after cat presentation, include movement arrest and risk assessment and the inhibition of non-defensive behaviors.

### Procedure:

1. The test apparatus for both the proxemics/activity and eat/drink procedures consists of two parallel subject chambers (53 × 20 × 25 cm).
2. Subject movements are monitored by five photocells mounted at equal distances.
3. The initial study assesses the effects of cat exposure on proxemics/activity, followed 7 days later analysis of eat/drink behavior during and after cat exposure. Both procedures are carried out under dim red light.

### Proxemic/activity testing:

1. Rats are individually placed in each compartment of the test apparatus. Following a 5- min pre-cat period, the cat is introduced to the cat compartment for 5 min. Following removal of the cat, behavior is recorded for a further 15 min post-cat period.

### Eat/drink testing:

1. Rats are individually given 2 g of finely crushed chocolate cereal on the 2 days after the proxemic/activity test, to familiarize them with this highly preferred food.
2. In order to induce a mild water deprivation, water bottles are removed, 24 h prior to eat/drink testing.
3. Same as proxemic/activity testing but measures of eating frequency and duration, and drinking frequency are taken for the cat and post-cat periods.

### Evaluation:

- The data are analyzed by analysis of variance (ANOVA).

## VIVA-VOCE

### Q.1 Define Anxiety.

**Ans:** Anxiety is chronic condition characterized by an excessive and persistent sense of apprehension with physical symptoms such as sweating, palpitations, and feelings of stress.

### Q.2 Write down the types of anxiety.

**Ans: Types of anxiety:**

1) Generalized Anxiety Disorder
2) Panic Disorder
3) Phobic Disorders - Agoraphobia, Acrophobia, Aquaphobia
4) Obsessive-Compulsive Disorder
5) Post-Traumatic Stress Disorder

# Experiment No. 15

## Object: To study the local anesthetics by different methods.

## Introduction:

- Local anesthetics are used to block the nerve supply to a limited area and are used only for minor and rapid procedures.
- This should be carried out under expert supervision for regional infiltration of surgical site, nerve blocks and for epidural and spinal anesthesia.
- They are used in various techniques of local anesthesia such as:
    - Topical anesthesia (surface)
    - Topical administration of cream, gel, ointment, liquid, or spray of anesthetic dissolved in DMSO or other solvents/carriers for deeper absorption
    - Infiltration
    - Brachial plexus block
    - Epidural (extradural) block
    - Spinal anesthesia (subarachnoid block)
    - Iontophoresis

## Properties of ideal anesthetic agents:

- It should not irritate the tissue to which it is applied.
- It should not make any long-lasting changes on nerve structure.
- Its systemic toxicity should be minimal.
- It must be effective regardless of whether it is injected into tissue or applied locally on mucous membranes.
- The time of onset of anesthesia should be minimal.
- Duration of action must be sufficiently long to allow the procedure to be completed but not so long as to necessitate extended recovery.
- It should have enough potency to administer full anesthesia without supplementing additional concentrated solutions that are potentially damaging.
- It should not produce allergic reaction.
- It should be stable in solution and should spontaneously undergo biotransformation in the body.
- It should be sterile or capable of being sterilized by heat without deterioration.

## Some screening methods for local anesthetics for preclinical study:

### 1. Conduction anesthesia:

### A. Conduction anesthesia in the sciatic nerve of the frog:

#### Procedure:

1. Frogs (*Rana temporaria*) of either sex are used and are kept at 4 °C. The frog is decapitated with a pair of scissors. The skin is incised in the thigh region at both sides and the sciatic nerves are carefully exposed in the thigh, avoiding any stretching and injury of the nerve.
2. The frog is suspended on a vertical board. Small pieces of white cotton are soaked with different concentrations of the test preparations (between 0.05% and 1%) or the standard and placed gently around the sciatic nerve for 1 min.
3. Then the cotton swab is removed and the frog is placed with its extremities into a bath with 0.65% Nacl solution. This allows testing for duration and reversibility of the local anesthetic effect.
4. One side is used for the test preparation and the other for the standard (e.g., 0.25% butanilicaine). Every 3 min the frog is removed from the bath and the toes of the legs or the ankle joint are pinched three times with a small forceps.
5. The reflex contraction is abolished when conduction anesthesia is effective. The stimuli are repeated every 3 min until anesthesia vanishes. Two to 5 frogs are used for each concentration.

#### Evaluation:

Time of onset and duration of anesthesia are recorded for each concentration. Time-response and dose-response curves can be established.

### B. Conduction anesthesia in the sciatic nerve of the rat:

#### Procedure:

1. Male Wistar or Sprague Dawley rats weighing 125 to 175 g are used. The animal is suspended in a prone position by grasping the base of the tail and thoracic cage.
2. A hind limb is extended to its full length and the depression for needle insertion is located by palpation with the left index finger. The site of injection is the area under the skin at the junction of the biceps femoris and the gluteus maximus muscles.
3. The sciatic nerve is blocked in the mid thigh region with 0.2 ml of the drug solution administered by a 24 to 25-gauge needle attached to a 0.25 ml tuberculin syringe.

4. Usually a 1% solution of the test drug in 0.9% Nacl is used as a test solution. The other leg is used for a control drug (e.g., procaine or lidocaine).
5. Immediately after the injection, repeated checks of the digit of the foot and the walking behavior are performed.
6. In the normal foot, the digits are wide apart, while in the blocked leg the digits of the foot are close together. Also the successful block is evidenced by dragging of the leg and an inability of the animal to use the leg in walking up the inclined wire mesh cover of the cage.
7. After the time of block for each leg is noted, each animal is examined every 5 to 10 min in order to note the time of recovery.

### Evaluation:

From the data, averages for onset and duration of action are calculated, plus the frequency of blocks are noted. Using various doses of test compound and standard, dose-response curves can be established and potency ratios calculated.

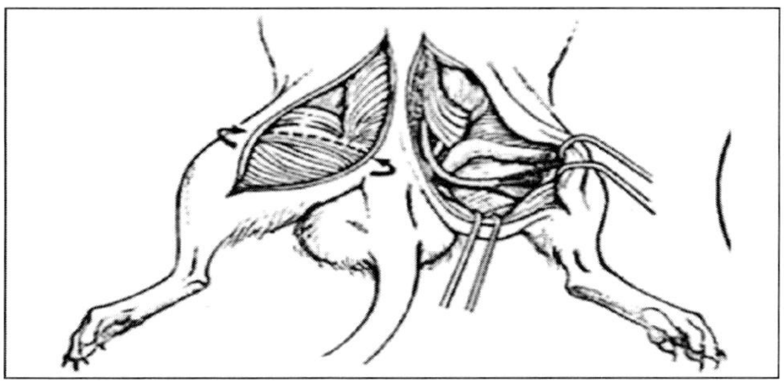

**Sciatic nerve of the rat**

## C. Conduction anesthesia on the mouse tail:

### Procedure:

1. Groups of 10 mice (NMRI-strain) of both sexes with a weight between 18 and 22 g are used for each dose. Before administration of the test compound or the standard the normal reaction time is determined.
2. The animal is placed into a small cage with an opening for the tail at the rear wall. The tail is held gently by the investigator. By opening of a shutter, a light beam exerting radiant heat is directed to the proximal third of the tail.
3. After about 6 sec, the reaction of the animal is observed by the investigator. The mouse tries to pull the tail away and turns the head. The shutter is closed with a switch when the investigator notices this reaction.

4. Mice with a reaction time of more than 6 sec are not used in the test. The test compounds and the standard are injected in a volume of 0.1 ml on both sides in the area of the tail root.
5. The animals are submitted to the radiant heat again after 10 min. The area of heating is about 1.5 cm distal to the injection site. For each individual animal the reaction time is noted.

### Evaluation:

There are two possibilities for evaluation:

i. The average values of reaction time after each time interval are calculated and compared with the pretest value by analysis of significance.
ii. At each time interval only those animals which show a reaction time twice as high or higher as the pretest value are regarded as positive. Percentages of positive animals are counted for each time interval and each dose and $ED_{50}$ values are calculated according to LITCHFIELD and WILCOXON.

## D. Retrobulbar block in dogs:

### Procedure:

1. Young female mongrel dogs weighing 13–15 kg are used. Twenty-four h before the test, 0.25% eserine (Physostigmine) ointment is placed in each conjunctival sac of the dog. Pentobarbital (25 mg/kg) is administered intravenously, then repeated with 10 mg/kg at hourly intervals, thus maintaining the animal in light anesthesia (corneal reflex present).
2. Ten min after induction, the dog is put into 30-degree head-down position, and 20 ml of 0.05% tetracaine is forced into the epidural space through the interarcuate ligament. Horner's syndrome occurs within 5 min.
3. A 150-watt surgical lamp is now focused upon the eye from 1 meter distance. 15 min later, a retrobulbar block is performed: The sclera is seized with an ophthalmic forceps and the eyeball is pulled downward and medially; a 23-gauge needle is then introduced through the superior rectus muscle, tangentially to the globe.
4. It is immobilized as soon as a click indicates penetration of the retrobulbar space; correct placement is confirmed by free motion of the needle tip and protrusion-rotation of the eyeball upon injection of 1 ml of air.
5. After aspiration, 2 ml of the tested anesthetic is then injected at a rate of 0.5 ml per second. The pupil dilates and reaches its maximal diameter (6 mm) within a few minutes.

6. This apparent diameter is estimated with a 2-cm long ruler calibrated in millimeters, whose center is gently applied to the corneal center.
7. The pupil is measured every 15 s for 5 min, then every 5 min until reappearance of maximal miosis (pinpoint and asymmetrical), a precise endpoint which generally coincides with corneal reflex and lacrimation.

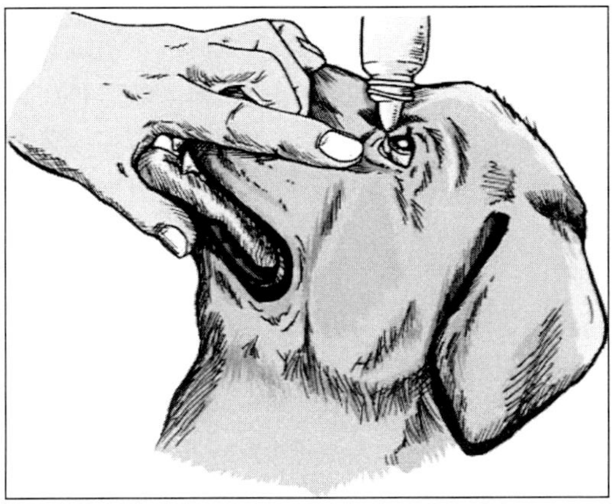

**Retrobulbar block in dogs**

### Evaluation:

Drug latency (in min) and duration (in 5-min units) are averaged for both eyes of each animal, and the mean and standard deviation then calculated for all test animals. Analysis of variance is performed to find significant differences between various local anesthetics.

## 2. Infiltration anesthesia:

### Procedure:

1. Adult guinea pigs of either sex weighing 250–300 g are chosen. On the day preceding the experiment the hair on the back is clipped and two areas of 4–5 cm diameter are shaved.
2. This produces a certain amount of irritation which disappears overnight. The sensitivity of the skin is greatest in the midline and slightly more so in the front than in the back area. For this reason each concentration of a local anesthetic must be tested in both areas.
3. Six tests using three guinea pigs can be performed simultaneously. The doses of local anesthetics are always injected intracutaneously in 0.1 ml saline. Three guinea pigs receive one dose in the front area and another dose in the back area; the size of the wheal is marked with ink.

4. One side is used for the test preparation, the other side for the standard (e.g., 1% butanilicaine).
5. The reaction to pin prick is tested 5 min after injection in the following way. After observing the animal's normal reaction to a prick applied outside the wheal, six pricks are applied inside the wheal and the number of pricks is counted to which the guinea pig fails to react.
6. The pricks are applied at intervals of about 3–5 s. Six pricks are applied every 5 min for 30 min. Having completed the test on 3 guinea pigs, the same solutions are injected into 3 other guinea pigs, but the solution which was used for the front is now used for the back area and vice versa.

### Evaluation:

- The number of times the prick fails to elicit a response during the 30 min period is added up, and the sum, out of possible 36, gives an indication of the degree of anesthesia.
- Using various doses, dose-response curves can be established. For time-response curves, the prick tests are repeated every 10 min. Half-life times are calculated as the time, when after complete anesthesia 3 out of 6 pricks elicit a response again.

## 3. Surface anesthesia:

## A. Surface anesthesia on the cornea of rabbits:

### Procedure:

1. Albino rabbits of either sex weighing 2.5–3 kg are placed into rabbit holding cages. The upper and lower eyelashes are carefully clipped.
2. The conjunctival sac of one eye is held open, thus forming a pocket. From a 1 ml syringe with a 22-gauge needle, 0.5 ml of a solution of the anesthetic is applied into the conjunctival sac for 30 s.
3. Then the procedure is repeated, so that 1.0 ml is applied within 1 min. One ml of the standard (0.1% solution of tetracaine hydrochloride) is applied to the other eye.
4. Effective local anesthetics extinguish the corneal reflex (blinking) elicited by any touch of the cornea. For quantitative purposes, the irritation with a bristle according to von Frey (1894, 1896, 1922) has been recommended.
5. An equine hair bending at a load of 230 mg is attached perpendicularly to a glass rod.
6. Within 25 s, the cornea is touched 100 times. The summation of many stimuli applied this way gives better results than a single touch with a glass rod. The test is started 5 min after application of the drug and repeated every 5 min until anesthesia vanishes and blinking occurs again. The time between disappearance and reappearance of the corneal reflex is registered.

### Evaluation:

Using the time of loss of the corneal reflex as parameter after application of different doses, dose-response curves can be established and potency ratios versus the standard calculated.

## B. Suppression of sneezing reflex in rabbits:

### Procedure:

1. Groups of male rabbits weighing 3 kg are used. Using a cotton tampon, the test solution is applied to the mucous membrane of one nostril.
2. The solution of a standard local anesthetic is administered to the nasal mucosa of the other nostril. After 2 min the mucous membrane is stimulated by a fine pencil. Loss of the sneezing reflex is regarded as sign of complete anesthesia.
3. The stimulation is repeated after 3, 6, 10 and 15 min and continued every 5 min until the sneezing reflex reappears. Various concentrations of test compound and standard are applied.

### Evaluation:

Using the loss of the sneezing reflex as parameter after application of different doses, dose-response curves can be established and potency ratios versus the standard calculated. Furthermore, the duration of activity can be evaluated.

## 4. Epidural anesthesia:

## Epidural anesthesia in guinea pigs:

### Procedure:

1. Male guinea pigs weighing 300–500 g are anesthetized by means of an intraperitoneal injection of an aqueous solution of chloral hydrate 42.5 g/l; ethanol 90 g/l; propylene glycol 428 g/l; sodium pentobarbitone 9.75 g/l; and magnesium chloride 21 g/l. A skin incision is made from the level of the lumbosacral fossa and approximately 1.5 cm down in order to expose the sacral area in the mid-line.
2. With the vertebral column flexed, the lumbosacral intervertebral ligament is carefully incised. Through this small opening a polyethylene catheter (PE 10) is inserted maximally 1.5 cm along the roof of the vertebral canal to the L4–L5 region.
3. The catheter is sutured to the overlying lumbar fascia which is then closed. The catheter is tunneled under the skin and exteriorized through an incision in the neck region.
4. After fixation of the catheter to the fascia of the neck muscles and suturations of the incisions, the catheter is filled with saline and sealed.

5. After a recovery period of at least 1 day, 0.1 ml of 2.0% lidocaine is injected over a period of 1 min, and the motor and sensory blocks are assessed.
6. The injection of lidocaine which results in a bilateral, reversible blockade indicates a successful preparation. A minimum of 8 animals are used in the further experiments for each test solution.

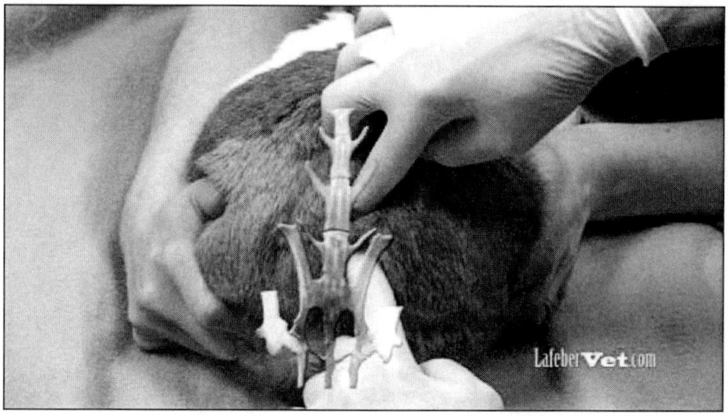


**Epidural anesthesia in guinea pigs**

### Evaluation:

Mean time to onset of block and mean duration of block are calculated from number of legs blocked.

## 5. Intrathecal (spinal) anesthesia:

### Spinal anesthesia in rats:

### Procedure:

1. Male Sprague-Dawley rats weighing 50–75 g are used. The rat is held firmly by the pelvic girdle. A 30-gauge needle is attached to a 25-μl Hamilton syringe is inserted into the tissue on one side of the L5 or L6 spinous process at an angle of about 20°.
2. The needle is advanced to the groove between the spinous and transverse processes and then moved forward to the intervertebral space at an angle of about 10°. About 0.5 cm of the needle is then in the vertebral column.
3. Correct placement of the needle is indicated by an arching of the tail. Drugs are dissolved in saline or water and administered in a volume of 5 μl.
4. Antinociception is determined in a modification of tail flick assay in rats by placing the tail of the rat under a focused radiant heat source.

## Evaluation:

- The degree of antinociception is defined as the percentage of maximum possible effect. This percentage is determined for each dose at each time measured allowing to calculate *ED*50 values.

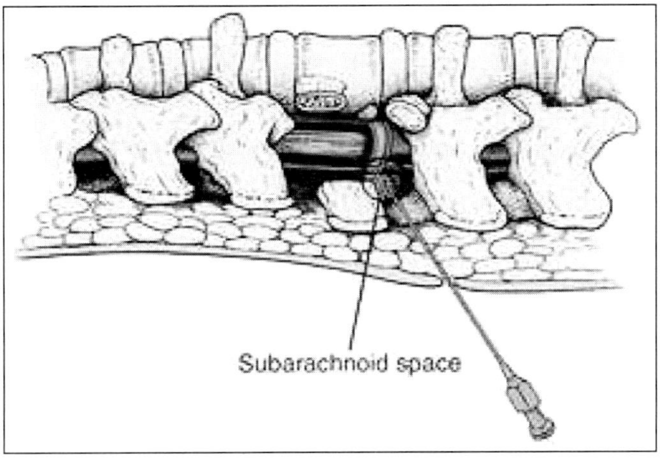


**Spinal anesthesia**

# VIVA-VOCE

**Q.1 Give the properties of ideal anaesthetic agents.**
**Ans: Properties of ideal anaesthetic agents:**

- It should not irritate the tissue to which it is applied.
- It should not make any long-lasting changes on nerve structure.
- Its systemic toxicity should be minimal.
- It must be effective regardless of whether it is injected into tissue or applied locally on mucous membranes.
- The time of onset of anesthesia should be minimal.
- Duration of action must be sufficiently long to allow the procedure to be completed but not so long as to necessitate extended recovery.
- It should have enough potency to administer full anesthesia without supplementing additional concentrated solutions that are potentially damaging.
- It should not produce allergic reaction.
- It should be stable in solution and should spontaneously undergo biotransformation in the body.
- It should be sterile or capable of being sterilized by heat without deterioration.

**Q.2 Give techniques of local anesthesia.**

**Ans: They are used in various techniques of local anesthesia such as:**

- Topical anesthesia (surface)
- Topical administration of cream, gel, ointment, liquid, or spray of anesthetic dissolved in DMSO or other solvents/carriers for deeper absorption
- Infiltration
- Brachial plexus block
- Epidural (extradural) block
- Spinal anesthesia (subarachnoid block)
- Iontophoresis

# Pharmacology-II

## (Semester-V)

# Experiment No. 1

## Object: To study the introduction of in-vitro pharmacology and physiological salt solutions.

## Theory:

### Introduction to *In-vitro* pharmacology:

Pharmacology is the study of the biological effects of drugs. In vitro pharmacology means studies on the biological effects of drugs and pharmaceuticals, conducted outside of living organisms. Any new drug or pharmaceutical that enters the market is a product of a long and rigorous development, testing, and approval process. At the early stage of drug discovery, the most promising molecules ("leads") undergo further screening to generate high-quality data in a precise and timely manner. All these parameters including chemical's safety, toxicity, pharmacokinetics, and metabolism must be assessed in the pre-clinical trials phase.

*In vitro* pharmacology studies are done in the laboratory. *In vitro* pharmacology includes study of therapeutic effects of a drug in an isolated environment, such as cell lines or tissues. This setup conveniently eliminates whole organism physiological influences allowing for a detailed analysis of a compound's impact.

"In vitro" is a latin word that means "within the glass" therefore the studies which are done outside the living organism, inside glass (test tubes or petridishes) are known as in vitro studies.

It is the experiment or observations done on the tissue outside of the living organism in a controlled environment, usually using petri dishes and test tubes.

In vitro processes, conditions are artificial and they are reconstructions of in-vivo environments. Artificial conditions are formed by mixing the necessary components and reagents under controlled conditions inside a glassware in the laboratory.

In vitro methods are widely used in Pharmaceutical industry to produce large scale pharamaceuticals using microorganism due to ease of production and economic benefits.

## Advantages of in-vitro studies:

- In vitro studies permit a species-specific.
- Simpler, more convenient
- More detailed analysis
- In vitro studies are replacing studies in whole animals.
- It is less expensive and provides quicker results.

## Disadvantages of in-vitro studies:

- The primary disadvantage of in vitro experimental studies is that it may be challenging to extrapolate from the results of in vitro work back to the biology of the intact organism.
- Investigators doing in vitro work must be careful to avoid over-interpretation of their results, which can lead to erroneous conclusions about organism and systems biology.
- A non-attendance of pharmacokinetics, in medicinal phrasing, is one of the critical downsides of *in vitro* pharmacological investigations. An absence of pharmacokinetics, just as a few different variables, can make it hard to extrapolate the outcomes to what may be normal when the medication is utilized in vivo.

## Physiological Salt Solutions (PSS):

Physiological salt solution can be defined as artificially prepared solution to keep isolated tissue alive under experimental conditions. They provide isotonicity, nutrition and act as a buffer when drugs are added. The physiological salt solutions are used to keep isolated tissue or organ preparations surviving as long as the experiment is over. It is important to choose the particular type of solution in which tissue is known to survive.

All physiological salt solutions are prepared in distilled water using analytical grade reagents. Physiological solutions are prepared fresh and used within 24 hours. Storage is not recommended because of the problems of microbial growth. While preparing the physiological salt solution, calcium chloride should be added last in the form of solution in order to prevent the precipitation of bicarbonate. Because isolated tissue will not survive for long periods in cloudy physiological salt solution. Cloudy physiological salt solution also gives erratic response with drugs. The other precautions to be taken are adjusting the proper pH of the final solution and aeration with oxygen, mixture of oxygen and carbondioxide (95%+5%) or even bubbling with air. The composition of physiological salt solution which are commonly used in the laboratory are given below.

**Table: Composition of Physiological Salt Solutions (PSS) (g/*l*):**

| Name of the ingredients | Name of the physiological salt solutions | | | | | | |
|---|---|---|---|---|---|---|---|
| | Ringer/ Ringer Locke | Frog Ringer | Tyrode | De Jalon | Kreb's-Henseleit | Mc Ewen | Hukovic |
| **NaCl** | 9.00 | 6.5 | 8.0 | 9.0 | 6.9 | 6.6 | 6.6 |
| **KCl** | 0.42 | 0.14 | 0.2 | 0.42 | 0.35 | 0.42 | 0.34 |
| **CaCl2** | 0.24 | 0.12 | 0.2 | 0.06 | 0.28 | 0.24 | 0.28 |
| **NaHCO3** | 0.5 | 0.2 | 1.0 | 0.5 | 2.1 | 2.1 | 2.1 |
| **MgCl2** | - | - | 0.1 | - | - | - | - |
| **MgSO4 • 7H2O** | - | - | - | - | 0.28 | - | - |
| **NaH2PO4** | - | 0.01 | 0.05 | - | - | 0.16 | - |
| **KH2PO4** | - | - | - | -- | 0.16 | - | 0.15 |
| **Glucose** | 1.0 | 2 | 1.0 | 0.5 | 2.0 | 2.0 | 2.0 |
| **Sucrose** | - | - | - | - | - | 4.5 | - |

## Following things should be carefully noted at the time of preparation of solution:

1. **Balance of ions:** Absolute quantity of each ion and preparation among each other especially with calcium and potassium must be maintained.
2. **pH of solution/reaction of solution:** pH of various PSS varies from 7.3-7.8 depending upon organ. At lower pH value, tone of preparations tends to decrease and impact of medicament is also altered. pH affects tissue directly and by ionization. At elevated pH, ionization is less and leads to alkalinity and thus improves cardiac and smooth muscle activity. During experiment there can be accumulation of metabolite which may change the pH. Buffering agents like $HCO_3$ and $PO_4$ are added in saline solution and solutions are changed frequently.
3. **Glucose:** Introduced by "Locke" and serves as source of energy, increases contractility of tissue. Glucose is not essential constituent for amphibian's tissue, but essential for mammalian tissues.
4. **Distilled Water:** Distilled water serves as a vehicle to dissolve various ingredients.
5. **Control of temperature:** For consistent effect, it is important to maintain the temperature of PSS, particularly for mammalian tissue. For instance, when temperature of solution is below 37°C, tone of intestine is decreased, increased contracts become smaller and contraction and relaxation time increases; whereas amphibian tissues survive for longer time in normal environment.

6. **Aeration:** Air, oxygen or oxygen + 5% carbon dioxide are required for the correct working of the tissues. Other than giving oxygen to the tissues, the flood of gas bubbles likewise blends the arrangements in the shower in this manner encouraging dissemination of the medications. The arrangement in the shower is ought to be changed oftentimes in light of the fact that delayed air circulation will in general modify pH.

## Use of each ingredient:

| S.No. | Ingredients | Use |
|---|---|---|
| 1. | Sodium Chloride (NaCl) | To maintain iso osmolarity,isotonicity,excitability and contractility of the preparation |
| 2. | Potassium Chloride (KCl) | To maintain ionic balance and responsible for increased relaxation of heart, increased neuromuscular transmission and excitability of nerves. |
| 3. | Calcium Chloride ($CaCl_2$) | To maintain the contractility of the preparation |
| 4. | Magnesium chloride and magnesium sulphate | Responsible for relaxation of smooth muscles. |
| 5. | Glucose | To provide energy |
| 6. | Sodium bicarbonate (NAHCO3) | To provide alkaline pH |
| 7. | Potassium dihydrogen phosphate or sodium dihydrogen phosphate | Acts as a buffer. |

## Different PSS and their uses:

| S.No. | PSS | Use |
|---|---|---|
| 1. | Ringer/Ringer Locke | For isolated rabbit heart perfusion |
| 2. | Frog Ringer | Used in rectus abdominis muscle, heart and other preparations of frog |
| 3. | Tyrode | For experimentation in rabbit intestine and guinea pig ileum, rat ileum, etc. |
| 4. | De-Jalon | Used in rat uterus etc. |
| 5. | Kreb's Henseleit | For tracheal chain of guinea pig, vas deferens, fundus strip of rat and aortic strip preparation of rabbit |
| 6. | Mc Ewen | Guinea pig seminal vesicles |

## Precautions:

1. Add sodium bicarbonate at the time of setting up of the experiment.
2. All the ingredients are accurately weighed.
3. Due to ppt formation, dissolve calcium chloride separately in distilled water in beaker.
4. Should always be prepared freshly in every experiment.

## VIVA-VOCE

**Q.1 Define PSS.**

**Ans.** Physiological Salt Solution can be defined as artificially prepared solution to keep isolated tissue alive under experimental conditions.

**Q.2 Enlist the various ingredients present in PSS.**

**Ans.** NaCl, KCl, CaCl2, NaHCO3, MgCl2, MgSO4•7H2O, NaH2PO4, KH2PO4, Glucose and Sucrose.

**Q.3 Give the uses of various PSS.**

**Ans.** **(i)** **Ringer Locke solution:** It is used in isolated rabbit heart perfusion.

**(ii)** **Frog Ringer solution:** Used in rectus abdominis muscle, heart and other preparations of frog.

**(iii)** **Tyrode solution:** For test of rabbit intestine and ileum of guinea pig, rat ileum etc.

**(iv)** **De-Jalon solution:** Used in rat uterus etc.

**(v)** **Kreb's Henseleit solution:** For tracheal chain preparations of guinea pig, vas deferens, fundus strips of rat and aortic strip preparation of rabbit.

**Q.4 Write significance of PSS.**

**Ans.** As experiments in animals are performed with isolated organs, it's essential to utilize a certain number of physiological solutions of different ionic concentration which almost operate like a substitute to the tissue fluid. They provide isotonicity, nutrition as well as work like a buffer when drugs are added.

**Q.5 Define *In vitro* pharmacology with advantage and disadvantage.**

**Ans.** ***In vitro* pharmacology** is the study finished in the laboratory and to study therapeutic outcomes of a drug in an isolated environment, such as cell lines or tissues.

**Advantages:** *In vitro* pharmacological investigations are significant in that they permit increasingly quick advancement of new medicines - numerous medications can be learned at once (and they can be contemplated in countless examples of cells) and just those that seem, by all accounts, to be strong go on to human examinations.

**Disadvantage:** A non-attendance of pharmacokinetics, in medicinal phrasing, is one of the critical downsides of *in vitro* pharmacological investigations. An absence of pharmacokinetics, just as a few different variables, can make it hard to extrapolate the outcomes to what may be normal when the medication is utilized in vivo.

# Experiment No. 2

## Object: To study the effect of drugs on isolated frog heart.

## Principle:

The drugs influence the rate (chronotropy) and force (inotropy) of contraction of the heart. An increase in the heart rate is called a "positive chronotropic" response, while a "negative chronotropic" response is a decrease in the heart rate. Similarly, an increase in the force of contraction is called a 'positive inotropic' response and a decrease in the force of contraction is called a 'negative inotropic' response. Heart is innervated by both sympathetic and parasympathetic nerves, which alter the basic rhythm of the heart and also that initiated by the pacemaker tissue of the SA node. Blood is supplied to the wall of the coronary arteries. Sympathomimetic amines such as adrenaline and noradrenaline produce positive inotropic and positive chronotropic response. Where as parasympathomimetics such as acetylcholine produce negative inotropic and negative chronotropic response.

## Requirements:

**Animal:** Frog

**Drugs:** Adrenaline (10μg/ml), Noradrenaline (10μg/ml), Acetylcholine (10μg/ml)

**Physiological salt solution:** Frog Ringer

**Equipments:** Heart lever, Sherrington's recording drum, Marriott's bottles, Syringe, needle Frog board.

## Procedure:

1. Set up the assembly.
2. Sacrifice the frog by pithing or by stunning.
3. Place the frog in a tray with ventral side facing up.
4. Make an incision to skin longitudinally and then expose the rectus muscle.
5. Make incision around the rectus muscle without damaging the frontal abdominal vein.
6. Expose the heart after cutting the sternum then pericardial membrane, remove and tie one part of aorta.
7. Put a knot around the inferior vena cava, then make a small cut for cannulation.

8. After cannulation with Syme's cannula, cut the other part of aorta and isolate the heart and perfuse with frog ringer solution. Supply frog ringer solution through the horizontal arm of the syme's cannula.
9. Place the heart clip on the heart apex, later connect it to a starling heart lever.
10. Record the normal heart beat on the drum.
11. Inject the graded doses of 0.05ml, 0.1ml, 0.2ml, 0.4ml, 0.8ml of adrenaline solution into syme's cannula. Immediately switch on the kymograph and record result of adrenaline for 2 minutes period. After 2 minutes turn off the kymograph till the heart beat and amplitude comes to normal.
12. Inject the graded doses of 0.05ml, 0.1ml, 0.2ml, 0.4ml, 0.8ml of noradrenaline solution into syme's cannula. Immediately switch on the kymograph and record result of noradrenaline for 2 minutes period. After 2 minutes turn off the kymograph till the heart beat and amplitude comes to normal.
13. Inject the graded doses of 0.05ml, 0.1ml, 0.2ml, 0.4ml, 0.8ml of acetylcholine solution into syme's cannula. Immediately switch on the kymograph and record the outcome of acetylcholine (ACh) for 2 minutes period. After 2 minutes turn off the kymograph till the heart beat and amplitude comes to normal.
14. Observe the onset and duration of action of all, i.e. adrenaline, acetylcholine, noradrenaline.

## Observation table:

| S.No. | Drugs | Dose (ml) | Effect of drug | | | | Result |
|---|---|---|---|---|---|---|---|
| | | | Force | Rate | Rhythm | Tone | |
| 1. | Adrenaline | | | | | | |
| 2. | Acetyl Choline | | | | | | |
| 3. | Noradrenaline | | | | | | |

## Precautions:

1. Remove the blood from the heart completely after giving the small cut (blood causes formation of clot and heart stops).
2. Give sufficient time for the heart to recover between the two doses of drug by taking the baseline every time.
3. The rotation of sherrington's recording drum should be away from the lever.

# VIVA-VOCE

**Q.1 What is action potential.**

**Ans.** A phenomenon of continuously varying potential difference across the cell membrane is called as action potential.

**Q.2 Define positive and negative chronotropic effect.**

**Ans.** An increase in the heart rate is called positive chronotropic effect, while negative chronotropic effect is a decrease in heart rate.

# Experiment No. 3

## Object: To study the effect of drugs on blood pressure and heart rate of dog.

## Principle:

The arterial blood pressure is defined as the pressure exerted by the blood on the walls of the blood vessels. Therefore, blood pressure = cardiac output × peripheral resistance. The heart and the blood vessels are under the control of autonomic nervous system.

Both sympathetic and parasympathetic nerves supply the heart. Parasympathetic innervation is through the vagus whereas the sympathetic nerve supply to the heart comes from fibres arising from stellate or inferior cervical ganglion. The nervous supply to the blood vessels are principally from the sympathetic system. In general, sympathetic stimulation (administration of adrenaline or noradrenaline) increases cardiac output and resistance to flow leading to an increased blood pressure.

On the other hand, parasympathetic stimulation (administration of acetylcholine) decreases cardiac output which lowers the blood pressure. Drugs which increase the blood pressure are called pressor agents, and those decrease are called depressor agent.

## Noradrenaline (NA):

It is a sympathomimetic catecholamine having predominate alpha receptor action. The effect of noradrenaline differs from that of adrenaline that rate is not increased. On the contrary it may decrease slightly. Only rise in blood pressure is seen and this is due to the vasoconstriction specially those which supply blood to skin and mucosa. Since beta action of NA is not seen, the effect of rise in blood pressure is more than adrenaline only.

## Adrenaline:

It is a sympathomimetic catecholamine which produces effect through alpha, beta1 and beta2 receptors. As a result of beta1 receptor stimulation there is sudden increase in heart rate and force of contraction and increase B.P. Immediately due to reflex inhibition there is slight decrease in B.P., but drug reaches to the periphery where alpha1 receptor stimulation produces vasoconstriction and hence, further rise in blood pressure is observed. A notch is seen due to sudden changes in the response. Adrenaline action is slowly terminated by reuptake and by monoamine oxidase (MAO) and catechol-o-methyl transferase

(COMT) enzymes. When the concentration of adrenaline is reduced beta2 receptor action predominates and as a result slight fall in blood pressure is seen.

## Isoprenaline:

It is a sympathomimetic amine which produces specific beta1 and beta2 receptor agonistic action. Beta1 receptors present in heart are excited by isoprenaline as a result of which there is increase in blood pressure and heart rate. When drug reaches periphery there occurs vasodilation of blood vessels specially which are supplied to skeletal muscle. As a result of this there is fall in blood pressure. Isoprenaline is not the substrate for uptake, hence, the termination of action takes time and there is delayed recovery.

## Acetylcholine:

It is a parasympathomimetic agent which can stimulate both muscarinic as well as nicotinic receptors. However, in low doses it produces only muscarinic receptor action and hence, there is fall in blood pressure due to dilatation of blood vessels. The action of Ach is rapidly terminated by cholinesterase enzyme and hence, the response of Ach gets quickly recovered. Heart rate does not change in response to Ach.

## Requirements:

**Animal**: Dog (6-8 kg)

**Drugs:** Adrenaline, noradrenaline, isoprenaline, acetylcholine (all 100 mg/ml stock solution), normal saline, and sodium citrate (10% w/v).

**Anaesthetic:** Pentobarbitone sodium (45 mg /kg, iv); prepare a stock solution containing 45mg/ml of the drug and per kg of body weight.

**Equipment:** Artery cannula, venous cannula, dog operating table, research kymograph (big), mercury manometer and surgical equipment.

## Procedure:

1. Anesthetise the dog with pentobarbitone (45 mg/kg) given intravenously.
2. Cannulate the femoral vein and connect it to a burette containing saline. Femoral vein cannulation is used for drug administration.
3. After that a midline incision is given in the neck skin and fascia is reflected, muscles are separated and trachea is exposed.
4. After exposing trachea search for the carotid artery, lying in the deeper tissue on the side of trachea.

5. An arterial cannula is inserted in the carotid artery and this cannula is connected to a mercury manometer with help of pressure rubber tubing.
6. This set is used for recording of blood pressure.
7. Record the base-line mean blood pressure response. Note the heart rate.
8. Inject 3 or 5 μg/kg adrenaline through the femoral venous cannula. Note the sequence of the response, i.e. rise in blood pressure, heart rate, the vagal notch, blood pressure falling below the base-line and recovery to pre-drug base line. Wait for 5-10 min.
9. Similarly administer noradrenaline, isoprenaline and acetylcholine, one after the other. Give sufficient gap (5-10 min) between the effect of two drugs.

## Precautions:

1. A healthy adult dog is given.
2. Anesthetic agent as per CPCSEA guidelines.
3. All the drugs concentration accurately given as per body weight.

## VIVA-VOCE

**Q.1 Define blood pressure.**

**Ans:** The arterial blood pressure is defined as the pressure exerted by the blood on the walls of the blood vessels.

**Q.2 Write down the formula of blood of pressure.**

**Ans:** Blood pressure = cardiac output × peripheral resistance.

# Experiment No. 4

## Object: To study the diuretic activity of drugs using rats/mice.

## Principle:

Diuretics are the compounds which increase the flow of urine. Normal urine output in rats is very small (1-2 ml/rat/day). Hence to get the measurable quantity the animals are first hydrated. The urine output is increased after administration of diuretics like urea, hydroflumethiazide and frusemide. Increase in volume of urine is measured with the help of measuring cylinder and compared with the normal urine output.

## Requirement:

**Animal:** Rats

**Equipments:** Metabolic cages and graduated measuring cylinder.

**Drugs and solutions:** Normal saline (0.9%), Urea (900 mg/kg; oral), Hydroflumethiazide (1mg/kg; oral), Frusemide (5mg/kg; oral)

## Procedure:

1. Albino rats (150-200 g) are fasted (deprived of food and water) overnight and saline (25ml/kg) is administered orally with the help of oral feeding cannula.
2. Those animals are divided into four groups containing three rats in each as follows:
   (i) Ist group- only normal saline (N.Saline)
   (ii) IInd group- saline + Urea (900 mg/kg; oral)
   (iii) IIIrd group-saline + hydroflumethiazide (1mg/kg; oral)
   (iv) IVth group-saline + frusemide (5mg/kg; oral)
3. After administration of drugs, animals are placed in four different metabolic cages.
4. Urine is collected in a measuring cylinder.
5. Time, when the first drop of urine is collected in a cylinder for each group is noted and the volume is recorded at intervals of 15 min for 3-4 hrs.
6. The difference in the volume collected at different time interval and total volume can be compared with various diuretics.

## Observation Table:

| S.No. | Groups | Amount of urine (ml) | | | | | | Total volume of urine (ml) |
|---|---|---|---|---|---|---|---|---|
| | | After 15 min | After 30 min | After 45 min | After 60 min | After 2 hr | After 3hr | |
| 1. | Group I | | | | | | | |
| 2. | Group II | | | | | | | |
| 3. | Group III | | | | | | | |
| 4. | Group IV | | | | | | | |

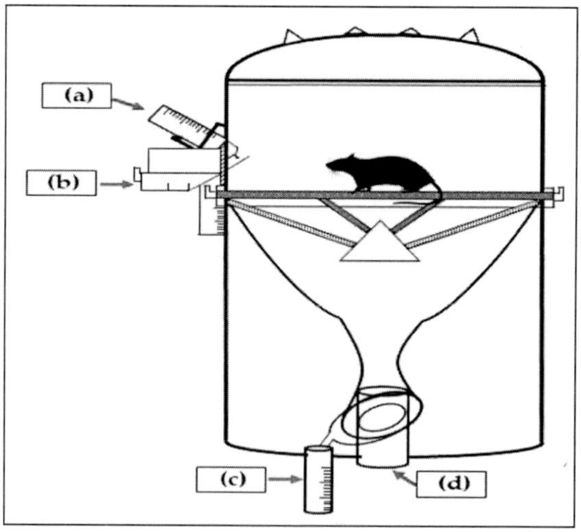


**Metabolic Cage**

## Precautions:

1. Selection criteria of drugs.
2. Specific strains of rats/mice selection.
3. Carefully total volume can be compared with various diuretics.

## VIVA-VOCE

**Q.1 Define diuretics.**

**Ans:** Diuretics are the compounds which increase the flow of urine.

**Q.2 Normal urine output in rats is:**

**Ans:** 1-2 ml/day

# Experiment No. 5

## Object: To study the Dose Response Curve (DRC) of acetylcholine using frog rectus abdominal muscle.

## Principle:

Frog rectus abdominal muscle is a voluntary muscle. At the neuromuscular junction, a nerve impulse liberates acetylcholine from the nerve ending into the cleft between muscle and nerve fiber. This acetylcholine causes a depolarization of the muscle fiber which in turn sets off a muscle action potential, and contraction of the muscle fiber. The muscle fibers of lower species like frog are multiply innervated and hence nerve stimulation causes persistent depolarization and a prolonged slow contraction of the muscle. Local administration of acetylcholine also produces similar effect. Frog rectus abdominal muscle contains nicotinic ($N_2$) receptors. Acetylcholine acts as an agonist.

Dose (concentration)-response curves demonstrate graded responses to drugs or agonists where an increase in response is recorded with a subsequent increase in the dose or the concentration of the drug. The dose–response curve is sigmoid or S- shaped. The first part (25% of graph) of the curve has poor discrimination between the doses whereas the middle portion of the curve shows greater sensitivity to different concentrations, and the responses to increasing concentrations are linearly differentiated. The last of the curve (plateau) shows the ceiling effect where no more increase in the response is seen with further increase in the dose.

When the doses are increased in geometric progression (logarithmic intervals) and the response is plotted against logarithms of doses, the relationship is called log dose-response curve.

The study of concentration or dose response curve indicates: (1) relative potency of the drug or agonist, when the curve is more towards the left, it indicates that the drug is more potent. The vice-versa is also true; and (2) slope of the curve indicates error and reliability (precision) of the bioassay. Steeper the slope more precise is the assay and vice versa is also true.

## Requirements:

**Animals:** Frog

**Drugs:** Acetylcholine stock solution (1mg/ml)

**Physiological solution:** Frog Ringer

## Procedure:

1. Pith or stun the frog and lay it on its back on the frog-dissecting board. Pin the four limbs.
2. Remove the skin on the abdomen and expose the rectus abdominal muscle.
3. Cut and prepare two rectus muscle preparations from each frog.
4. Tie a thread to the top and bottom of each muscle preparation before detaching the muscle from the body of the frog.
5. Mount the preparation in up-right position in the organ bath containing frog Ringer solution under a tension of 1 g. There is no need of maintaining the bath temperature since it is an amphibian tissue preparation. Bubble the organ with air.
6. Relax the tissue for 45 min, during which period wash the tissue with fresh quantum of ringer for at least four times.
7. Record the concentrations due to acetylcholine using either simple sideway or frontal writing lever. 90 second contact time and a total 5 min time cycle may be used for proper recording of the responses.
8. Record at least four responses to increasing doses of acetylcholine or till you get the maximum response. The maximum response is achieved if one gets same or slightly less response with a higher concentration. Properly label the graph, put the date, your name, and fix the tracing with the help of fixing solution.
9. Measure the height of the response (mm) and draw a dose (concentration)- response graph.

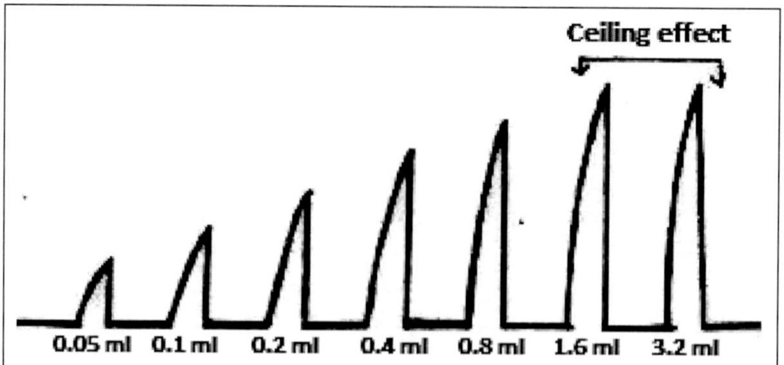


Dose Response Curve (DRC) of Ach

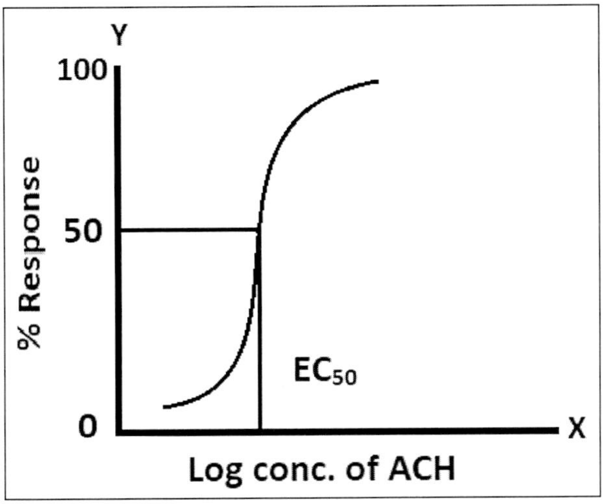


**Dose Response Curve (DRC) of Ach**

## Observation Table:

| S.No. | Dose of acetylcholine (ml) | Concentration (µg) | Log concentration | Response height (mm) | % Response height |
|---|---|---|---|---|---|
| 1. | 0.1 | 100 | 2 | | |
| 2. | 0.2 | 200 | 2.301 | | |
| 3. | 0.4 | 400 | 2.602 | | |
| 4. | 0.8 | 800 | 2.903 | | |
| 5. | 1.6 | 1600 | 3.204 | | |
| 6. | 3.2 | 3200 | 3.505 | | |

## Precautions:

1. Cut out all the blood capillaries present on muscle preparation by using a sharp scissor.
2. Use thin piece of muscle (2-3cm) as it is more sensitive than bulky piece.
3. The level of ringer solution in the organ bath should remain constant throughout the experiment by marking the level with elastic ring/marker.
4. Speed of the drum should be slow (0.25mm) and the lever should be placed tangential to the drum.
5. The no. of washing and the interval between them should be kept constant.

## VIVA-VOCE

**Q.1 Define DRC.**

**Ans:** Dose (concentration)-response curves demonstrate graded responses to drugs or agonists where an increase in response is recorded with a subsequent increase in the dose or the concentration of the drug. The dose–response curve is sigmoid or S- shaped.

**Q.2 Define log dose-response curve.**

**Ans:** When the doses are increased in geometric progression (logarithmic intervals) and the response is plotted against logarithms of doses, the relationship is called log dose-response curve.

# Experiment No. 6

## Object: To record the effect of physostigmine on the concentration response curve of acetylcholine using isolated rectus abdominal muscle preparation of frog.

### Principle:

Physostigmine is an anticholinesterase substance and it inhibits the metabolic break-down of acetylcholine. As a result the action of acetylcholine is potentiated. The concentration response curve of acetylcholine will be shifted to the left in the presence of physostigmine.

### Requirements:

**Animals:** Frog

**Drugs:** Acetylcholine stock solution (1mg/ml), Physostigmine stock solution (1 mg/ml)

**Physiological solution:** Frog Ringer

### Procedure:

1. Pith or stun the frog and lay it on its back on the frog-dissecting board. Pin the four limbs.
2. Remove the skin on the abdomen and expose the rectus abdominis muscle.
3. Cut and prepare two rectus muscle preparations from each frog.
4. Tie a thread to the top and bottom of each muscle preparation before detaching the muscle from the body of the frog.
5. Mount the preparation in up-right position in the organ bath containing frog Ringer solution under a tension of 1 g. There is no need of maintaining the bath temperature since it is an amphibian tissue preparation. Bubble the organ with air.
6. Relax the tissue for 45 min, during which period wash the tissue with fresh quantum of ringer for at least four times.
7. Record the concentrations due to acetylcholine using either simple sideway or frontal writing lever. 90 second contact time and a total 5 min time cycle may be used for proper recording of the responses.
8. Record at least four responses to increasing doses of acetylcholine or till you get the maximum response. The maximum response is achieved if one gets same or slightly less response with a higher concentration.

9. Add physostigmine (2µg/ml) to the reservoir containing frog ringer and irrigate the tissue with eserinised Ringer for 30 min.
10. Repeat the concentration response curves of acetylcholine in the presence of physostigmine.
11. Label and fix both the concentration response curves of acetylcholine, i.e. one in the absence and the other in the presence of physostigmine. Note the potentiation in the response of acetylcholine and calculate the relative $EC_{50}$ values.

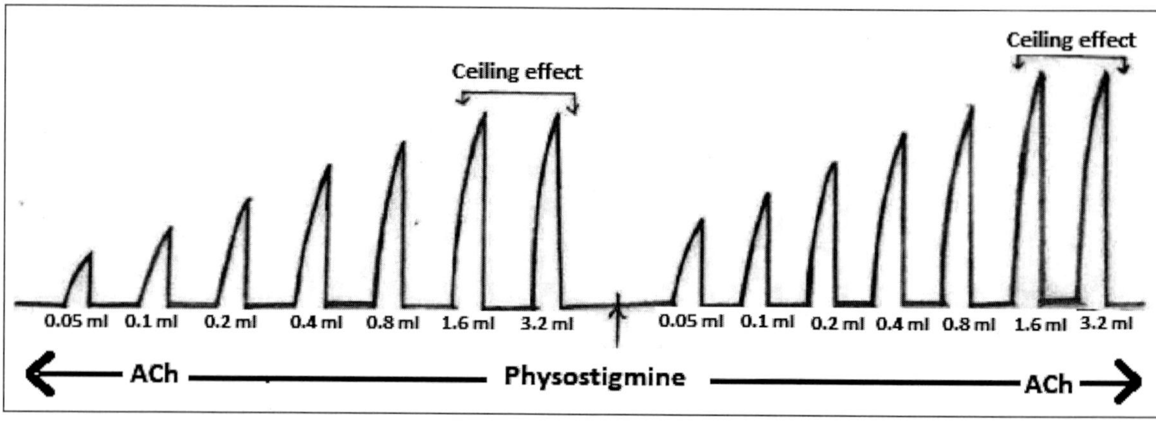


**Effect of physostigmine on the concentration response curve of acetylcholine**

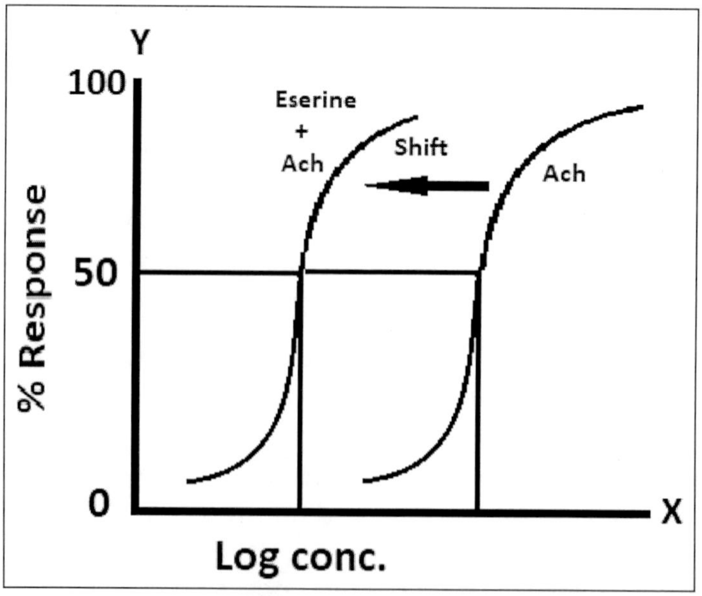


**Concentration response curves of acetylcholine in the presence of physostigmine.**

## Observation Table:

| S.No. | Dose of acetylcholine (ml) | Concentration (μg) | Log concentration | Response height (mm) without physostigmine | % Response height |
|---|---|---|---|---|---|
| 1. | 0.1 | 100 | | | |
| 2. | 0.2 | 200 | | | |
| 3. | 0.4 | 400 | | | |
| 4. | 0.8 | 800 | | | |
| 5. | 1.6 | 1600 | | | |
| 6. | 3.2 | 3200 | | | |

| S.No. | Dose of acetylcholine (ml) | Concentration (μg) | Log concentration | Response height (mm) with physostigmine | % Response height |
|---|---|---|---|---|---|
| 1. | 0.1 | 100 | 2 | | |
| 2. | 0.2 | 200 | 2.301 | | |
| 3. | 0.4 | 400 | 2.602 | | |
| 4. | 0.8 | 800 | 2.903 | | |
| 5. | 1.6 | 1600 | 3.204 | | |
| 6. | 3.2 | 3200 | 3.505 | | |

$$\textbf{Dose ratio} = \frac{EC_{50} \text{ in the presence of serine}}{EC_{50} \text{ before eserinization}}$$

## Precautions:

1. The level of ringer solution in the organ bath should remain constant throughout the experiment by marking the level with elastic ring/marker.
2. Speed of the drum should be slow (0.25mm) and the lever should be placed tangential to the drum.
3. The no. of washing and the interval between them should be kept constant.

## VIVA-VOCE

**Q.1 Define antagonism.**

**Ans:** The relationship between drugs in which an antagonist inhibits the activity of an agonist by reacting with the receptor or other part of the effector mechanism.

**Q.2 What is the action of physostigmine in presence of acetylcholine.**

**Ans:** Physostigmine is a competitive and non-competitive substance and it inhibits the metabolic break-down of acetylcholine.

**Q.3 What is the effect of physostigmine of isolated abdominal muscle of frog.**

**Ans:** Physostigmine is an anticholinesterase substance and it inhibits the metabolic break down of acetylcholine.

# Experiment No. 7

## Object: To demonstrate competitive antagonism between acetylcholine and atropine on rat ileum.

## Principle:

Rat ileum is an intestinal smooth muscle. Acetylcholine causes the contraction of the smooth muscle by acting on muscarinic receptors. Atropine blocks muscarinic receptors in the smooth muscle. Therefore, atropine blocks acetylcholine induced contraction in rat ileum. The concentration response curve of acetylcholine will be shifted to right in the presence of atropine. The nature of antagonism is of competitive type and thus surmountable.

The spontaneous contractions of the preparation can be reduced by reducing the calcium content in physiological salt solution and maintaining the bath at room temperature.

## Requirements:

**Animals:** Rat

**Drugs:** Acetylcholine (10 µg/ml), Atropine (1 µg/ml)

**Physiological solution:** Tyrode

**Conditions:** Temperature: 37°C

Tension: 0.5gm

Magnification: 10 times

Aeration: 70-72 Bubble/min

## Procedure:

1. The assembly is set up and arrangements are made for experimental conditions mentioned above.
2. Rat which is fasted overnight is sacrificed as per CPCSEA recommended guidelines.
3. The abdominal cavity is quickly opened and a piece of ileum is isolated.
4. It is placed in a petri dish containing tyrode solution maintaining at 37°C.
5. Mount the preparation in up-right position in the organ bath containing tyrode solution under a tension of 0.5 g.

6. Relax the tissue for 45 min, during which period wash the tissue with fresh quantum of tyrode for at least four times.
7. Record the concentrations due to acetylcholine using frontal writing lever. 90 second contact time and a total 5 min time cycle may be used for proper recording of the responses.
8. Record at least four responses to increasing doses of acetylcholine or till you get the maximum response. The maximum response is achieved if one gets same or slightly less response with a higher concentration.
9. Add atropine (1µg/ml) to the reservoir containing tyrode and irrigate the tissue with atropinised tyrode for 30 min.
10. Repeat the concentration response curves of acetylcholine in the presence of atropine.
11. Label and fix both the concentration response curves of acetylcholine, i.e. one in the absence and the other in the presence of atropine. Calculate the relative $EC_{50}$ values and note the nature of antagonism.

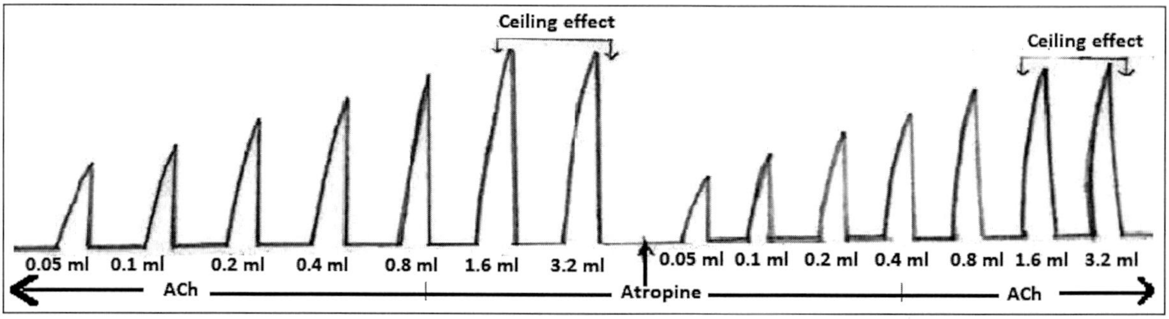


**Effect of atropine on the concentration response curve of acetylcholine**

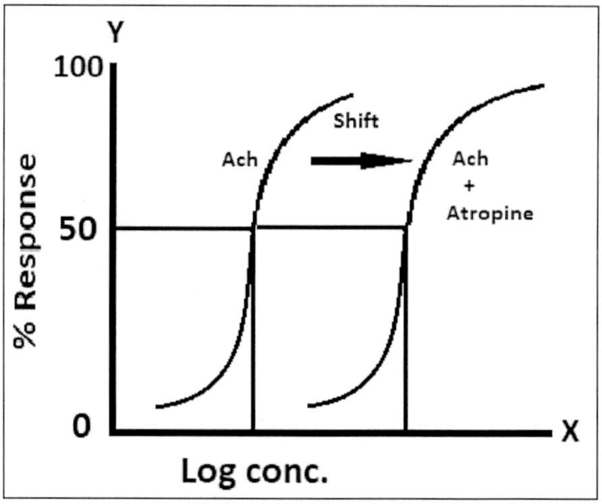


**Concentration response curves of acetylcholine in the presence of atropine.**

## Observation Table:

| S.No. | Dose of acetylcholine (ml) | Concentration (µg) | Log concentration | Response height (mm) without atropine | % Response height |
|---|---|---|---|---|---|
| 1. | 0.1 | 100 | 2 | | |
| 2. | 0.2 | 200 | 2.301 | | |
| 3. | 0.4 | 400 | 2.602 | | |
| 4. | 0.8 | 800 | 2.903 | | |
| 5. | 1.6 | 1600 | 3.204 | | |
| 6. | 3.2 | 3200 | 3.505 | | |
| | | | | | |
| **S.No.** | **Dose of acetylcholine (ml)** | **Concentration (µg)** | **Log concentration** | **Response height (mm) with atropine** | **% Response height** |
| 1. | 0.1 | 100 | 2 | | |
| 2. | 0.2 | 200 | 2.301 | | |
| 3. | 0.4 | 400 | 2.602 | | |
| 4. | 0.8 | 800 | 2.903 | | |
| 5. | 1.6 | 1600 | 3.204 | | |
| 6. | 3.2 | 3200 | 3.505 | | |

$$\textbf{Dose ratio} = \frac{EC_{50}\text{ in the presence of atropine}}{EC_{50}\text{ before atropine}}$$

## Precautions:

1. The level of ringer solution in the organ bath should remain constant throughout the experiment by marking the level with elastic ring/marker.
2. Speed of the drum should be slow (0.25mm) and the lever should be placed tangential to the drum.
3. The no. of washing and the interval between them should be kept constant.

## VIVA-VOCE

**Q.1 What is action of atropine in presence of acetylcholine.**

**Ans:** Atropine is a competitive antagonist of the actions of acetylcholine and other muscarinic agonists. Cardiac muscle muscarinic receptors are blocked. Muscarinic receptors in exocrine glands smooth and ganglia and intramural neurons are also blocked by atropine.

**Q.2 Define antagonism.**

**Ans:** The relationship between drugs in which an antagonist inhibits the activity of an agonist by reacting with the receptor or other part of the effector mechanism.

**Q.3 Write down the formula of dose ratio.**

**Ans:**

$$\textbf{Dose ratio} = \frac{\textbf{EC}_{50}\ \textbf{in the presence of atropine}}{\textbf{EC}_{50}\ \textbf{before atropine}}$$

# Experiment No. 8

## Object: To study the introduction to Bioassay.

## Theory:

Bioassay may be defined as the determination of the concentration of a biologically active substance, of physical, chemical or biological origin, by using a biological indicator with reference to standard. Bioassay is comparative in nature.

Bioassay is the determination or estimation of the amount of biological activity in a unit quantity of the preparation. It is a process of determining relative potency of a substance or active principle of a substance by comparing its biological activity with that of a reference standard. Bioassay includes both quantitative assays of drugs as well as the application of qualitative biological tests. The purpose of bioassay is to determine the potency of a drug and hence it serves as the quantitative part of any screening procedure. Other purpose of bioassay is to standardize the preparation so that each contains uniform specified pharmacological activity.

## Biological indicator:

The biological activity of a substance can be studied by using different experimental animals, isolated tissues of the experimental animals, immune cells or microorganisms are termed as biological indicator.

## Biological standardization:

Comparison and adjustment of the strength of the unknown sample with that of the standard under rigidity controlled conditions is termed as bio-standardization. It is a process of increasing or decreasing the potency of a biologically active substance to match it with the biological activity of a reference standard. Matching of material of unknown potency with an international/national standard objective of providing a reliable preparation for the use in therapeutics research. For example, matching of LD50 of digitalis tincture (which contain variable quantities of the active principle) to the standard preparation.

## Principles of Bioassay:

The basic principle of bioassay is to compare the test substance with the international standard preparation of the same and to find out how much test substance is required to produce the same biological effect, as produced by the standard. The following are the principles of bioassay:

1. All bioassays (lab studies, toxicity studies, clinical studies) must be comparative & compared against a standard drug or preparation. The potency of biologically assayed compounds is compared with the activity of internationally accepted standards.
2. The standard and new drugs should be as far as possible identical to each other, then their dose response curve (DRC) will have the same stop and would be constant all along the response level.
3. The biological response should be closely related to the therapeutic use of the drug as possible. For example, in estimating the potency of insulin, blood glucose levels would be of the ideal index, but the method commonly used is the mouse convulsion method, in which the % of animals developing convulsions are recorded. Similarly for estimating digitaloid drug, the arrest of heart in pigeon or guinea pig is used as end point which is as the toxic effect of the drug and not the therapeutic effect.
4. An estimate of relative potency is made by comparing the log dose of the test and the log dose of the standard that produces an equal magnitude of effect.
5. The problem of biological variation must be minimized as far as possible. For that one should keep uniform experimental conditions and assure the reproducibility of the responses. The results of the test should be subjected to statistical analysis to minimize errors due to biological variations.

## Applications of bioassay:

1. To standardize drugs of natural origin, especially when the chemical identity of the active has not been elucidated fully. e.g: parathyroid hormones, antitoxins etc.
2. To standardize those drugs from which no adequate chemical assay has been devised even though the chemical structure of the active principle has been established.e.g. Hormones like insulin, oxytocin etc.
3. To standardize the drugs which are composed of a complex mixture of substances with varying structure and activity. e.g: digitalis, posterior pituitary extract etc.
4. If the chemical assay is not a valid indication of the biological activity, e.g. due to lack of differentiation between active and inactive isomers.
5. To standardize when the drugs have same pharmacological actions but different chemical structures existing together. e.g: glycosides in digitalis preparation.
6. To estimate the dose of a drug required to produce a therapeutic or toxic response. e.g: calculation of ED50, LD50 etc.

7. When the physical property of rotation (dextro or levo) shows difference in action. e.g: d- Chloramphenicol is active. Levo adrenaline is 80 times more active than dextro.

## Types of bioassay:

Bioassay may be broadly classified into two types depending upon the type of response recorded i.e. i) quantal bioassay and ii) graded bioassay.

### (i) Quantal bioassay:

Quantal means the response is in the form of "all or none", i.e. either maximum response or no response. In this type of bioassay, there is no intermediate response. For example animal receiving a convulsant drug either show convulsions or does not. Examples of drugs assayed by quantal bioassay method are:

**Digitalis:** by cardiac arrest in guinea pig or pigeon.

**d-Tubocurarine:** by rabbit head drop method.

**Insulin:** by hypoglycaemic convulsions produced in mice.

Though the method is not very accurate, it is employed for comparison of threshold response and comparison of ED50 or LD50 values. The quantal bioassay is an end point method.

### End point method:

Here the threshold dose showing a positive effect is measured on each animal and the comparisons between two groups of animals are done i.e. one receiving standard and other the test compounds. e.g. bioassay of digitalis in cats. Here the cat is anaesthetized with chloralose and its blood pressure is recorded. The drug is slowly infused into the animal and the moment the heart stops beating and blood pressure falls to zero, the volume of fluid infused is noted down. Two groups of animals, one using standard digitalis and the other using test preparation of digitalis and then potency is calculated as follows:

$$\text{Concentration of unknown} = \frac{\text{Threshold dose of standard}}{\text{Threshold dose of test}} \times \text{Concentration of standard}$$

### (ii) Graded bioassay:

Graded response means the response is proportional to the dose and response may lie between no response and the maximum response. These responses are based on the observations that there is a proportionate increase in the observed response with a subsequent increase in the concentration or dose. This procedure depends on the precision of assay demand, quality of the sample available, availability of experimental animals.

### Types of graded assay are:

(a) Matching
(b) Bracketing
(c) Interpolation
(d) Multiple point bioassay (three point, four point, six point, eight point).

### (a) Matching Method:

It is the most simple type of bioassay. In this type of bioassay the response of the test substance is taken first and the observed response is tried to match with the response that is obtained with the standard drugs. Several responses of standard drug are recorded till a close matching response to that of test substance is observed. A corresponding concentration is thus calculated. This assay is employed when the sample size is very small. Since the assay does not involve the recording of concentration response curve, the sensitivity of the preparation is not taken into consideration. Therefore, the precision and reliability are not very good by this method.

### (b) Bracketing Method:

This method is made use of when the test sample is small. It is also a simple assay procedure. The response due to test substance is bracketed between two responses (greater and smaller) of standard substance. The precision and reliability of this procedure is also poor. Initially, two responses of the standard are taken. The doses are adjusted such that one is giving response of approximately 20% and other 70% of the maximum. The response of unknown which lies between two responses of standard dose is taken. The panel is repeated by increasing or decreasing the doses of standard till all three equal responses are obtained. The dose of test sample is kept constant. At the end, a response of the double dose of the standard and test which match each other are taken. These should give equal responses. Concentration of the test sample can be determined as follows:

$$\text{Concentration of unknown} = \frac{\text{Dose of standard}}{\text{Dose of test}} \times \text{Concentration of standard}$$

### This method has following limitations:

1. It occupies a larger area of the drum as far as tracings are concerned.
2. There are chances of errors that one cannot determine.
3. It does not give any idea of dose-response relationship.
4. The precision and reliability of this assay procedure is poor.

### (c) Interpolation Method:

In this type of bioassay a concentration-response curve of a standard substance is first established. Then record 2-3 responses due to test substance. The selection of the test responses should be such that they lie on the linear portion of the concentration response curve of the standard drug. It is a simple method and chances of errors are less if the sensitivity of the preparation is not changed. The precision and reliability of the assay is much better as compared to matching assay as the sensitivity of the preparation is assessed prior to testing the unknown sample.

### (d) Multiple point bioassay:

In this bioassay, the responses are repeated several times and the mean of each is taken. Thus, chances of error are minimized in these methods. The sequence of responses is recorded as per the Latin square method of randomization in order to avoid any bias.

### Three point bioassay:

This method is also based on the assumption of dose-response relationship. At first, the concentration response curve due to graded doses of a standard substance followed by the dose response curve of the test substance is recorded. Then, two standard doses and one test dose are selected from the respective DRCs such that they lie on the straightest and steepest part of the DRC. The test dose is selected in such a way that its response is greater than that of smaller dose of standard and is lesser than that of larger dose of the standard.

Bioassay is then carried out with the chosen standard and the test doses in 3 successive cycle as per the Latin square design. The responses are recorded in the order of

- $S_1, S_2, T$
- $S_2, T, S_1$
- $T, S_1, S_2$

The height of contraction of all the standard and test doses in the bioassay is measured. Then, a log DRC is plotted with the mean values of the standard responses in the bioassay and the dose of the standard producing the same response as produced by the test sample is directly read from the graph and the concentration of the test sample is determined. The concentration of the unknown can also be determined mathematically as follows;

Concentration of unknown = $n_1/t \times \text{anti log} \{T\text{-}S_1 / S_2\text{-}S_1 \times \log n_2/n_1\}$ Cs

n1 = Lower Standard dose
n2 = Higher Standard dose
t = Test dose
S1 = Response of n1

S2 = Response of n2
T = Response of test (t)
Cs = Concentration of standard

**Four point bioassay:**

This method is almost similar to the three point bioassay, but in this method 2 doses of the standard and the 2 doses of the test are used. The section of the standard doses should be such that they lie on the linear portion of the CRC and also the ratio between the smaller to greater dose should be preferably 1:2. The selection of the test doses is done by hit and trial method so that the responses fall on the linear part of the curve. By employing the latin square design, the responses of the chosen standard and the test doses is recorded in 4 successive cycles, in the order of

- $S_1, S_2, T_1, T_2$
- $S_2, T_1, T_2, S_1$
- $T_1, T_2, S_1, S_2$
- $T_2, S_1, S_2, T_1$

The height of contraction of all the standard and test doses in the bioassay is measured and their mean values are calculated. The concentration of the test sample can be determined by graphical method as well as mathematically by employing the following formula:

Concentration of unknown = $n_1/t_1 \times \text{anti log}\ \{(S_1+S_2)-(T_1+T_2)/(S_2+T_2)-(S_1+T_1) \times \log n_2/n_1\}$

n1 = Lower Standard dose
n2 = Higher Standard dose
$t_1$ = Lower Test dose
$t_2$ = Higher test dose
S1 = Response of n1
S2 = Response of n2
$T_1$ = Response of test ($t_1$)
$T_2$ = Response of test ($t_2$)

The precision, reliability and reproducibility of this assay method is very high. Hence, it is the most commonly used bioassay for the estimation of the concentration of active substances present in the biological fluids.

## Bioassay of Antagonists:

Commonly used method for the bioassay of antagonist is simple graphical method. The responses are determined in the form of the percentage inhibition of the fixed dose of agonist. These are then plotted against the log dose of the antagonist and the concentration of unknown is determined by finding out the amount of standard producing the same effect as produced by the test.

In this method, two responses of the same dose of agonist (sub maximal giving approximately 80% of the maximum response) are taken. The minimum dose of standard antagonist is added in the bath and then the response of the same dose of agonist is taken in presence of antagonist. The responses of agonist are repeated every ten min till recovery is obtained. The higher dose of standard antagonist is added and responses are taken as before. Three to four doses of the standard antagonist are used and then one to two doses of test sample of the antagonist is used similarly. The percentage inhibition is calculated, plotted against log dose of antagonist and the concentration of unknown is determined as usual.

## Advantages:

1. A chemical assay finds out only the amount of active substance present in a given sample where as the bioassay measures the actual biological activity of the active substance.
2. Bioassay measures small traces of compound too.
3. Bioassay can establish the biological activity of a substance even when its chemical identity is not known.
4. Sensitivity of a bioassay is greater than a chemical assay.
5. Chemical unstable drugs can be conveniently assayed by a bioassay.
6. The active and the inactive isomers present in a racemic mixture can be easily distinguished by a bioassay.

## Disadvantages:

1. Complicated set up.
2. Expensive.
3. Time consuming.
4. Too laborious
5. Requires skilled labor.
6. The effect observed in animals may not be observed in humans.
7. The quantitative accuracy of a bioassay usually falls considerably below that attainable with most chemical assays.

## Bioassay of Some Important Drugs:

Depending upon pharmacological action of various drugs, different preparations may be used. Following chart gives different preparations and the pharmacological activity for which a particular drug is assayed:

| Drugs | Preparation | Activity Assayed |
|---|---|---|
| Digitalis | Cat blood pressure | Fall in B.P. and death |
| | Guinea pig blood pressure | Stoppage of heart and death. |
| | Pigeon | Emesis |
| Adrenaline | Blood pressure of the spinal cat | Rise in B.P. |
| | Isolated rabbit duodenum, Isolated caecum of fowl, Isolated rat uterus | Inhibition of the tone |
| Noradrenaline | Blood pressure of the pithed cat | Rise in B.P. |
| Acetylcholine | Isolated rectus abdominis muscle of frog, Rat ileum and Leech dorsal muscle | Contractile effect. |
| | Isolated mouse heart | Inhibition of cardiac Contractions |
| | Rat/Cat blood pressure | Fall in blood pressure |
| Histamine | Isolated, atropinized terminal ileum of guinea pig. | Contractile effect |
| | Anaesthetized and atropinized cat. | Fall in blood pressure |
| 5-Hydroxy-tryptamine | Isolated atropinized rat uterus, Isolated terminal colon of rat, Isolated fundus strip of rat stomach. | Contractile effect |
| | Perfused rabbit ear | Constriction of blood vessels |
| Curariform drugs | Rabbit | Dropping of head |
| e.g. d-tubocurarine | Rat diaphragm with phrenic nerve | Inhibition of contractile effect |
| Heparin | Ox with thrombokinase extract and acetone dried ox brain | Prolongation of blood clotting time |
| Antibiotics | Suitable micro-organism grown on suitable nutrient agar medium | Inhibition of growth of micro-organism |
| Vitamin D | Rats maintained on richetogenic diet | Alleviation of rachetic stage. |

| Drugs | Preparation | Activity Assayed |
|---|---|---|
| Insulin | Rabbits | Lowering of blood-sugar Level. |
| | Mice | Convulsions and/or death due to hypoglycaemia |
| | Isolated rat diaphragm | Increase in glycogen content. |
| | Rat's epididymal fat | Increased metabolism of glucose, indicated by increase in $CO_2$ production. |
| Oxytocin | Adult cockerel | Vasodepressor activity. |
| | Isolated rat uterus | Contractile effect |
| | Rabbits (female) | Ejection of milk from mammary duct. |
| Vasopressin | Rat blood-pressure | Vasopressor activity. |
| Growth hormone | Hypophysectomized | Hypophysectomized |
| | Rats | Increase in width of epiphysea cartilage |
| Gonadotrophin (FSH) | Hypophysectomized male rats | Increase in testicular weight. |
| | Hypophysectomized female rats | Increase in ovaries weight |
| Gonadotrophin (L.H.) | Immature male rats | Enlargement of prostate gland. |
| Gonadotrophin (FSH and LH) | Immature female rats | Increase in weight of uterus. |
| *Prolactin | Cloves of pigeons sac. | Increase in weight of crop |
| | Female g. pig or rabbit. | Secretory changes in mammary gland. |
| | Female rats | Lengthening of estrous cycle and function of corpus luteum |
| | Hypophysectomized rat | Inhibition of estrogen upon vaginal smear. |
| *Corticortrophin | Hypophysectomized rats | Depletion of ascorbic rats acid from adrenal gland. |
| *Thyrotropin | Mice or rats | Release of previously administered 131I (Iodine) from thyroid gland |

| Drugs | Preparation | Activity Assayed |
|---|---|---|
| *Androgen | Castrated capon | Increase in size of comb. |
| | Castrated male rat | Increase in weight of prostate gland and seminal vesicles. |
| | Castrated male rats | Increase in weight of levator-animuscles |
| Estrogen | Rat or mouse | Increase in weight of (Female) uterus |
| Progesterone | Sexual immature rabbits | Proliferative changes in endometrium of uterus Increase in carbonic anhydrase-activity in uterus |

***Radioimmunoassay or radio receptor assay methods are also available.**

## (i). Bioassay of acetylcholine

**Principle:** Potency of the test sample is compared with that of the standard preparation. There are several biological methods for its assay.

**1. Rectus Abdominis Muscle of Frog:** Dissect the rectus muscle and arrange the assembly as per assay of d-tubocurarine. Plot log dose-response curve and find out the potency of the sample of acetylcholine.

**2. Cat's Blood Pressure:** A cat is anaesthetized with suitable anaesthetic. The carotid artery is cannulated for recording BP. Femoral vein is cannulated for injecting acetylcholine. Trachea is cannulated for giving artificial respiration. Acetylcholine produces a fall in BP by dilating peripheral blood vessels. This principle is utilised for its bioassay. The extent to which BP falls due to the test sample is compared with the fall by the standard preparation.

**3. Guinea-pig Ileum:** Guinea–pig is killed by a blow on the head and bled to death. The abdominal wall is dissected out so as to isolate the ileum, the faecal matter, mesentery and bood vessels are removed from the piece of ileum. It is ligated on both sides and suspended in mammalian organ bath containing Tyrode solution maintained at 37.0oC and oxygenated continuously. Acetylcholine contracts the ileum. This principle is utilised for its bioassay. The extent of contraction produced by the test sample is compared with the standard preparation of acetylcholine.

**4. Anaesthetised Rats:** Compare the extent of fall in BP of the test sample with that produced by the standard preparation.

**5. Leech Muscle:** Compare the contractions produced by the standard and test samples on eserinised dorsal muscle of the leech. This muscle is highly sensitive (picograms) to acetylcholine.

**6. Isolate Heart Preparations:** Rabbit's auricle, frog's heart, rabbit's heart or venous merceneria's heart is used. Ach decreases the force and rate of the heart.

**7. Rabbit's Intestine and Tracheal Chain:** Ach contracts these tissues.

## (ii) Bioassay of adrenaline

**Principle:** Potency of the test sample is estimated by comparing the rise in blood pressure of the test sample with that produced by the standard preparation of adrenaline.

**Standard Preparation:** It should fulfill all the tests of purity as per adrenaline monograph in the Indian Pharmacopoeia. The specific rotation of 4% w/v solution of the standard adrenaline in 0.1 N HCl should lie between –5 oC to 5 oC dilutions of adrenaline are prepared by diluting it with saline. A suitable concentration is 1: 10,000. Test sample solution is also prepared in saline.

**1. Method using Anaesthetised Dog:** A medium size dog (10-13 kg) is anaesthetised with pentobarbitone sodium in a dose of 25 mg/kg, i.v. Artificial respiration is given through tracheal tube, if necessary. BP is recorded on a kymograph after cannulating carotid artery with arterial cannula and connecting the same with a mercury manometer.

The animal should be given 0.001-0.002 mg of atropine sulphate to paralyse the vagi. This paralysis is confirmed by stimulating vagi by electrical stimulation. There will be no fall in BP in atropinised animal after electrical stimulation.

Adrenaline is injected into the femoral vein through venous cannula. Two successive responses of the same dose of adrenaline are noted. The similar responses after the same doses of adrenaline, is an indication that there is no variation in B.P., and that the animal is now ready for the assay. Then the test and the standard samples are given in alternate till both produce similar rise in BP. Injections are given at intervals of five minutes. Potency of the test sample is compared with that of the standard sample.

**2. On Spinal Cat:** Refer pressor activity of posterior pitutary extract and apply the same method.

**3. Method Using Rabbit's Duodenum:** A rabbit weighing 2-3 kg is killed by headblow method and bled to death. The animal is dissected out, the abdominal organs are exposed to isolate the duodenum. The duodenum is suspended in the inner bath of the mammalian organ bath.

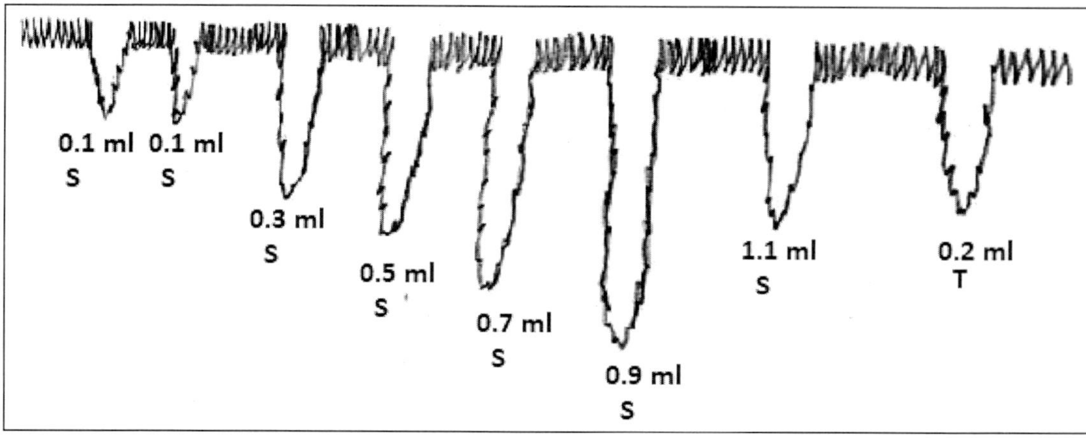


Inner bath is filled with Tyrode solution which is maintained at 37.5 oC. The muscle is allowed to stabilize for 30 min. Rhythmic contractions are recorded by means of the isotonic frontal writing lever on the kymograph. Adrenaline relaxes the duodenum and the same property is taken upto consideration for finding out the potency of the test sample. Adrenaline is bioassayed by graphical method as shown in Fig. 5.

**4. De Jalon's Method on Rat's Uterus:** This method was first demonstrated by De Jalon. A virgin female rat, weighing about 100-150 g is used for the experiment. The rat is killed by the headblow method and bled to death. The abdomen is opened and uterine horns are isolated and placed in a petri dish containing de Jalon solution. Uterine horns are ligated and suspended in a mammalian organ bath containing modified Ringer solution having the following composition is used:

NaCl 9.0 gm; CaCl2 0.06 gm; KCl 0.45 gm; Dextrose 0.5 gm NaHCO3 0.5 gm and distilled water 1000 ml. This solution abolishes the rhythmic contraction of the uterus. It is maintained at 37oC and bubbled continuously with air.

Two identical contractions for 30 sec with carbachol are recorded (0.75 mcg/ml). Then selecting three different doses of standard adrenaline and one intermediate dose test adrenaline the percentage reduction of carbachol induced contractions are recorded.

**5. Straub's Method:** In this method, a glass cannula is passed through the aorta and valves into the ventricle of heart so that the solution is pumped up and down in the cannula with every beat. A graph paper attached behind the cannula to give an estimate of the force of contraction of systole of the heart at every beat. The beat is recorded by attaching the tip of the ventricle through a thread to a lever. This preparation has been widely use for the detection of small quantity of adrenaline. Adrenaline increases the force of contraction of the ventricle. The increased force produced by the test sample is compared with that of the standard preparation.

## (iii). Bioassay of D-Tubocurarine

**1. Rabbit Head-drop Method : Principle:** d-Tubocararine hydrochloride is injected into the marginal vein of a rabbit's ear till the rabbit's neck muscles are relaxed such that the animal cannot hold its head up. The total amount of test sample required to produce the endpoint is compared with the total amount of the standard sample required to produce similar endpoint.

**Selection of Rabbits:** Rabbits weighing 2 kg are used. Animals should be free from disease, obtained from a healthy colony and should be accustomed with the experimental procedure.

**Experimental Procedure:** Each rabbit is placed in a holder with its head protruding outside. The head should be freely movable. Minimum 8 rabbits are used. They are divided into two groups each containing 4 rabbits. First group will receive standard sample and the second group will receive the sample under test. d-Tubocurarine solution is injected at a constant speed by infusion apparatus through the marginal vein.

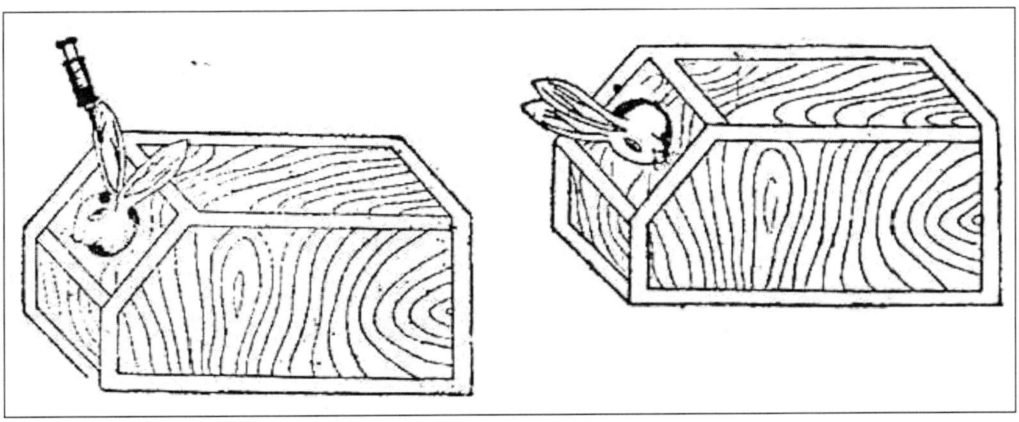

**Figure: Rabbit head drop method for the bioassay of d-tubocurarine.**
(i) i.v. inj. of d-tubocurarine. (ii) Head drop after injection.

Injection should be given at a rate of 0.4 ml/min and should take about 10 min. Infusion is continued till the rabbit will not be in a position to hold its head erect or there will be no response by focussing light on the eyes and the neck gets elongated and toneless.

Suitable dose of d-tubocurarine is 0.012% w/v in saline. Rabbits recover immediately from the effect of curarization. During the expt. there is a possibility of respiratory embarrassment which is treated by injecting neostigmine methyl sulphate (0.05 mg.) and atropine sulphate immediately through the marginal ear vein.

Cross-over test is carried out to minimise biological error due to animal variation. Those rabbits which received the standard sample on the first day will be given test sample on the second day of expt. and vice versa. Mean dose which produces head drop of the test sample is compared with the mean dose of standard preparation.

**2. Frog's Rectus Abdominis muscle Preparation:** A frog is pithed and laid on its back on a cork covered board to which it is pinned. The skin covering the abdomen is cut away and the rectus abdominis muscle of one side is dissected from the pelvic girdle to its insertion in the cartilage of the pectoral girdle. The muscle is then pinned to the cork by four pins to keep its normal length while a thread is sewn through each end. It is then mounted in the organ bath containing frog's Ringer solution which contains : NaCl, 6.5gm; KCl, 0.29 gm; CaCl2, 0.24 gm; NaHCO3, 0.4 gm; glucose, 1.5 gm and distilled water 2000 ml. Oxygenation is carried out to keep the tissue alive. The muscle is stabilized for 30-45 min. in order to get critical quantitative response. The responses are recorded using isotonic frontal writing lever with 1 G tension.

Two similar contractions with the same concentration of acetylcholine are obtained. Three doses of the standard sample and one intermediate dose of the test sample are selected and the reduction in height of contraction induced by acetylcholine is noted down.

Acetylcholine contraction is recorded on slow moving drum for 90 sec. d-Tubocurarine is allowed to act for 30 sec. The percentage reduction at each dose levels is calculated and log dose response curve of the standard drug is plotted. A linear response will be obtained. The potency of test sample is calculated from the standard curve.

## (iv). Bioassay of digitalis

**Principle:** Potency of the test sample is compared with that of the standard preparation by determining the action on the cardiac muscle. Any other equivalent method, which gives results similar to those obtained by this method are also valid.

**Standard Preparation and Units:** The standard preparation is a mixure of dried and powdered digitalis leaves (1 unit = 76 mg.)

**Preparation of Extracts:** Exact amount of the powder is extracted with dehydrated alcohol in a continuous extraction apparatus for six hours. The final extract should contain 10 ml. (5 ml. alcohol + 5 ml. water) per 10 g. of digitalis powder. It should be stored in between 5°C and –5°C.

**1. Guinea–pig Method (End point method):** Standard and test sample extracts are diluted with normal saline in such a way that 1 g of digitalis powder is diluted to 80 ml. A guinea pig is anaesthetized with a suitable anaesthetic. It is dissected on the operation table. The jugular vein is traced out by removing adhering tissues and cannulated by means of venous cannula. A pin is inserted in the heart, such that it gets inserted in the apex of the heart. In this way, we can observe the heart beats by up and down movements of the pin. The injection is continued through venous cannula untill the heart is arrested in systole. The amount of extract required to produce this effect is taken as the lethal dose of the extract.

Another set of 19 animals of the same species are used for this experiment and the average lethal dose is determined. It is not necessary to determine the lethal dose of the std. during each time of the experiment. But it should be occasionally checked.

The lethal dose of the test sample is determined in a similar way using minimum 6 guinea–pigs of the same strain.

The potency of the test sample is calculated in relation to that of the std. preparation by dividing the average lethal dose of the sample to the test and expressed as units per gram.

**2. Pigeon Method:** Minimum 6 pigeons are used for testing each sample. They should be free from gross evidence of disease or emaciation. The weight of the heaviest pigeon should not exceed twice the weight of the lightest pigeon. Food is withheld 16-28 hours before the experiment. Pigeons are divided on the basis of their sex, weight and breed, into two groups. They are anaesthetized with anesthetic ether.

One side of the wing is dissected and the alar vein is cannulated by means of a venous cannula. Dilutions are made with normal saline. Average lethal dose of each sample is determined; results are tabulated and calculated as per guinea pig method. The lethal dose per kg of body weight is determined for each pigeon. The potency of the test sample is determined by dividing the mean lethal dose of standard by the mean lethal dose of the test sample.

In pigeons, stoppage of heart is associated with a characteristic vomiting response called 'emesis'. The milk from the crop sac of pigeons is being ejected out. This may be taken as the end point response of digitalis.

## (v). Bioassay of insulin

**Standard preparation and unit:** It is pure, dry and crystalline insulin. One unit contains 0.04082 mg. This unit is specified by Ministry of Health, Government of India and is equivalent to international unit.

**Preparation of standard solution:** Accurately weigh 20 units of insulin and dissolve it in normal saline. Acidify it with HCl to pH 2.5. Add 0.5% phenol as preservative. Add 1.4% to 1.8% glycerin. Final volume should contain 20 units/ml. Store the solution in a cool place and use it within six months.

**Preparation of test sample solution:** The solution of the test sample is prepared in the same way as the standard solution described above.

**1. Rabbit Method: Selection of rabbits:** They should be healthy, weighing about 1800-3000 gm. They should then be maintained on uniform diet but are fasted for 18 hrs before assay. Water is withdrawn during the experiment.

**Standard and Sample Dilutions**: These are freshly prepared by diluting with normal NaCl solution so as to contain 1 unit/ml. and 2 units/ml.

**Doses**: The dose which can produce suitable fall in blood sugar level is calculated for the standard.

**Principle:** The potency of a test sample is estimated by comparing the hypoglycemic effect of the sample with that of the std. preparation of insulin. Any other suitable method can also be used.

**Experimental Procedure:** Animals are divided into 4 groups of 3 rabbits each. The rabbits are then put into an animal holder. They should be handled with care to avoid excitement.

**First part of the Test:** A sample of blood is taken from the marginal ear vein of each rabbit. Presence of reducing sugar is estimated per 100 ml. of blood by a suitable chemical method. This concentration is called 'Initial Blood Sugar Level'.

The four groups of rabbits are then given sc. injections of insulin as follows:

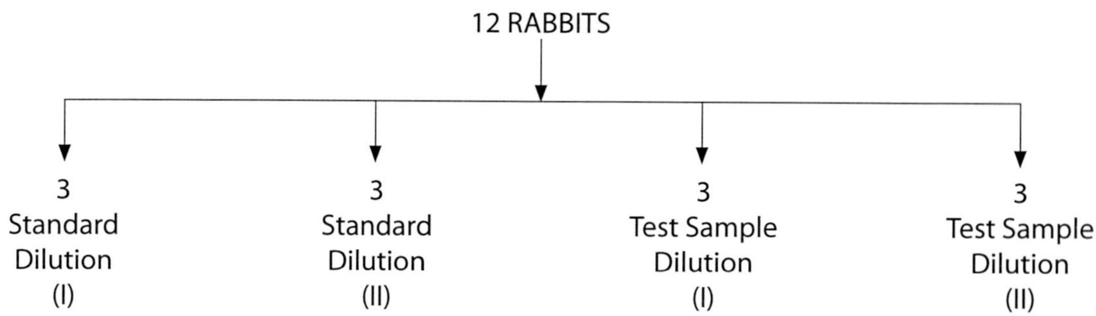


From each rabbit, a sample of blood is withdrawn up to 5 hrs at the interval of 1 hr. each. Blood sugar is determined again. This is known as 'Final Blood Sugar Level'.

**Second part of the test (Cross over test):** The same animals are used for the second part. The experiment can be carried out after one week. Again they are fasted and initial blood sugar is determined. The grouping is reversed, that is to say, those animals which received the standard are given the test and those which received the test are now given the standard. Those animals which received the less dose of the standard are given the higher dose of the test sample and vice-versa. This test is known as 'Twin Cross Over Test'.

Mean percentage decrease in blood sugar of the first and second part is calculated.

**2. Mouse Method:** Mice show characteristic convulsions after s.c injection of insulin at elevated temperatures. The percentage convulsions produced by the test and standard preparations are compared.

**Experimental procedure**: Minimum 100 mice weighing between 18-22 gm of the same strain are used. They should be maintained on constant diet. They should be fasted 18 hrs prior to the experiment.

**Standard and sample dilutions:** Dilutions are prepared with sterile saline solution, so as to contain 0.064 units/ml. (std dilution I) and 0.096 untis/ml. (std. dilution II). Similarly, test sample solutions are also prepared.

Mice are divided into 4 groups each containing 25 mice and insulin is injected s.c as follows:

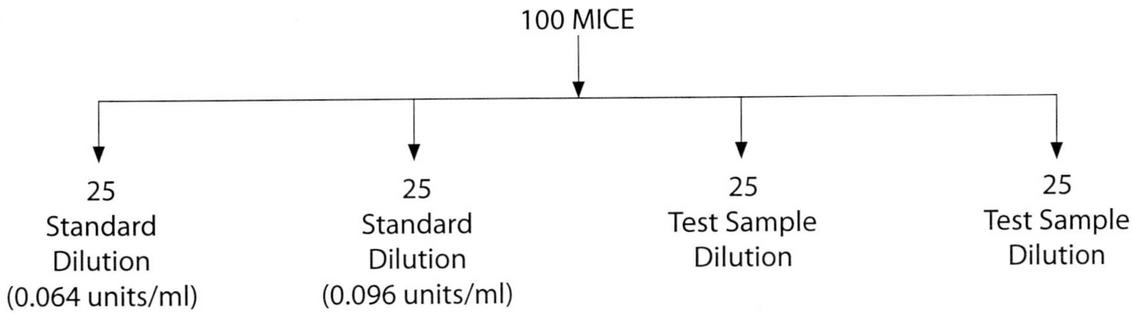


Mice are put in an air incubator at 33oC and observed for one and a half hr. An air incubator with a glass front provided with six shelves is used. The temperature is thermostatically controlled. Two mice are kept in each of the boxes made up of perforated sheets of metal.

The mice which convulse or die are taken out of the incubator and observed. These mice usually convulse severely but failure of the animal to upright itself when placed on its back, should as well be considered as convulsion. Convulsive mice may be saved by an inj. of 0.5 ml. of 5% dextrose solution.

Percentage convulsions produced by the test sample are compared with those of the standard sample. Those animals which survive may be used again for another expt. after an interval of one week.

| Dose | S1 0.25 ml | S2 0.25 ml | T1 0.25 ml | T2 0.25 ml |
|---|---|---|---|---|
| Convulsions | | | | |
| Percentage Convulsions | | | | |

**3. Rat diaphragm method:** In this method increase in glycogen content of the muscle or increase in glucose uptake by muscle in response to insulin is taken as the index of potency of insulin.

**4. Rat epididymal fat-pad method:** Here, the ability of insulin to increase $CO_2$ production by the fat-pad is taken as the parameter for the measurement of potency of the insulin preparation.

**5. Radioimmunoassay:** It is the estimation of the concentration of the substance in a unit quantity of preparation using radiolabelled antigens. A number of drugs are estimated now days by radioimmunoassy methods because these methods are highly specific and highly sensitive.

The radioimmunoassay of insulin is based on the ability of human insulin (unlabelled) to displace beef's insulin (which may be labelled) from the binding sites (i.e. antibodies). The method involves the following steps:

I. Bovine insulin is injected into the sheep. After a week the serum containing antibodies produced against bovine insulin is collected form the blood of the sheep.
II. The serum containing antibodies is exposed to radiolabelled insulin and the bound vs free ratio is determined.
III. The mixture of labelled antigen-antibodies is then added in different test-tubes labelled as standard and test. About 6 concentrations of the standards are taken. They are then added to different tubes and the bound vs free ratio is again determined using gamma-counter.
IV. Standard curves are determined and the concentration of test insulin is determinded using this standard curve.

## (vi). Biological Assay of Heparin Sodium

**Principle:** The potency of heparin sodium is determined by comparing the concentration necessary to prevent the clotting of sheep or goat or human plasma with the concentration of the Standard Preparation of heparin sodium necessary to give the same effect under the conditions of the following method of assay.

**Standard Preparation and Unit**: The Standard Preparation is the freeze-dried sodium salt of the purified active principle from bovine intestinal mucous membranes or any other suitable preparation, the potency of which has been determined in relation to the International Standard. The Unit is the specific activity contained in 7.7 μ g of the Standard Preparation and is the same as the International Unit; 1 mg contains 130 Units.

**Special Reagents: Prepared Plasma:** Collect blood from sheep or goats or human volunteers directly into a vessel containing 8% w/v solution of sodium citrate in the proportion of 1 volume to each 19 volumes of blood to be collected. Mix immediately by gentle agitation and inversion of the vessel. Immediately centrifuge and pool the separated plasma. To 1 ml of the pooled plasma in a clean test-tube add 0.2 ml of a 1% w/v solution of calcium chloride and mix. The plasma is suitable if a solid clot forms within 5 minutes.

**Solution of standard preparation:** Determine by preliminary trial, if necessary, approximately the minimum quantity of the Standard Preparation of heparin sodium which, when added in 0.8 ml of saline solution, maintains fluidity in 1 ml of prepared plasma for 1 hour after the addition of 0.2 ml of a 1% w/v solution of calcium chloride. On the day of the assay prepare a solution of the Standard Preparation such that it contains in each 0.8 ml of saline solution the above-determined quantity of the Standard Preparation.

**Test solution:** Weigh accurately about 25 mg of the preparation being examined and dissolve in sufficient saline solution to give a concentration of 1 mg per ml and dilute to a concentration estimated to correspond to that of the solution of the Standard Preparation.

**Method:** To very clean test-tubes (150 mm x 16 mm) add graded amounts of the solution of standard preparation, selecting the amounts so that the largest dose does not exceed 0.8 ml and so that they correspond roughly to a geometric series in which each step is approximately 5% greater than the next lower. To each tube add sufficient saline solution to make the total volume 0.8 ml. Add 1.0 ml of prepared plasma to each tube. Then add 0.2 ml of a 1% w/v solution of calcium chloride, note the time, immediately stopper each tube with a suitable stopper and mix the contents by inverting three times in such a way that the entire inner surface of the tube is wet.

In the same manner set up a series using the test solution, completing the entire process of preparing and mixing the tubes of both the solution of standard preparation and the test solution within 20 minutes after the addition of the prepared plasma. Exactly one hour after the addition of the calcium chloride solution, determine the extent of clotting in each tube, recognizing three grades between zero and full clotting.

The dilution of the test solution which contains heparin sodium in the same concentration as the dilution of the solution of standard preparation is that contained in the series of dilutions which show the same degree of clotting as the series of dilutions of the solution of standard preparation. If the degree of clotting observed in the series of dilutions of the solution of standard preparation lies between that observed in two of the series of dilutions of the sample being examined, the potency of the latter is estimated. If there is no such correspondence between the degrees of clotting produced by the solution of standard preparation and any of the dilutions of the sample being examined, new dilutions of the latter are prepared and assay is repeated.

Carry out no fewer than three independent assays. Calculate the estimated potency of the preparation being examined by combining the results of these assays by standard statistical methods.

Limits of error - The limits of error (P = 0.99) attainable with the test are:

90 and 110%, with three determinations;
92 and 108%, with four determinations.

Heparin Sodium intended for use in the manufacture of injectable preparations without a further procedure for the removal of pyrogens complies with the following additional requirement.

## (vii). Biological Assay of Oxytocin

**Principle:** The potency of oxytocin is determined by comparing its activity with that of the Standard Preparation of oxytocin under the conditions of a suitable method of assay.

**Standard Preparation**: The Standard Preparation is the 4th International Standard for Oxytocin, established in 1978, consisting of freeze-dried synthetic oxytocin peptide with human albumin and citric acid (supplied in ampoules containing 12.5 Units), or another suitable preparation the potency of which has been determined in relation to the International Standard.

### Suggested methods

**Method A**: **By depression of the blood pressure in chicken** — Anaesthetise a young healthy adult cockerel weighing 1.2 to 2.3 kg with an anaesthetic that will maintain a prolonged and constant high blood pressure. Expose the gluteus primus muscle in one thigh and cut and retract it to reveal the popliteal artery and crural vein. Cannulate the popliteal artery and record the blood pressure on a suitable recorder calibrated for use over a linear range. Cannulate the crural or brachial vein. Immediately before use prepare a solution of the Standard Preparation in saline solution so that the volume to be injected is between 0.1 ml and 0.5 ml. Record the blood pressure responses to the injection into the cannulated vein of two doses of this solution; the doses should be such as to produce clearly discriminated, precipitous, submaximal decreases in blood pressure; the required doses normally lie between 20 and 100 milliUnits. The interval between injections should be constant and lie between 3 and 10 minutes depending on the rate at which the blood pressure returns to normal. Immediately before use dilute the preparation being examined with saline solution so as to obtain responses similar to those obtained with the Standard Preparation. The ratio between the two doses of the preparation being examined should be the same as that between the two doses of the Standard Preparation and this ratio should be kept constant throughout the assay.

The two doses of the Standard Preparation and the two doses of the preparation being examined should be given according to a randomised block or a Latin square design and at least six responses to each should be recorded.

If the animal rapidly becomes insensitive to the repeated injections of the solutions another animal must be used. Measure all the responses and calculate the result of the assay by standard statistical methods.

**Method B**: **By contraction of the rat uterus** — Inject 100 mcg of oestradiol benzoate intramuscularly into a female rat weighing 120 to 200 g 18 to 24 hours before the assay. Immediately before the assay confirm by vaginal smear that the rat is in oestrus or preoestrus. Kill the rat and suspend one horn of the uterus in a bath containing a solution of the following composition:

| Composition (% w/v) | |
|---|---|
| Sodium chloride | 0.662 |
| Potassium chloride | 0.045 |
| Calcium chloride | 0.007 |
| Sodium bicarbonate | 0.256 |
| Disodium hydrogen phosphate | 0.029 |
| Sodium dihydrogen phosphate | 0.003 |
| Magnesium chloride | 0.010 |
| Dextrose | 0.050 |

Maintain the bath at a temperature of 32° or at some other suitable temperature at which spontaneous contractions of the uterus are abolished and the preparation maintains its sensitivity. Oxygenate the solution with a mixture of 95% of oxygen and 5% of carbon dioxide and record the contractions of the muscle using a suitable instrument giving a linear response (for example an isotonic lever with a load not exceeding 2 g). Record the ontractions produced by the addition to the bath of two doses of the Standard Preparation suitably diluted with the above solution. The doses should be such as to produce clearly discriminated, submaximal contractions; the required doses normally lie between 10 and 50 micro Units per ml of bath liquid. When maximal contraction has been reached, replace the bath liquid by a fresh solution. The doses should be added at regular intervals of 3 to 5 minutes depending upon the rate of recovery of the muscle. Dilute the preparation being examined so as to obtain responses on the addition of two doses similar to those obtained with the Standard Preparation. The ratio between the two doses of the preparation being examined should be the same as that between the two doses of the Standard Preparation and this ratio should be kept constant throughout the assay.

The two doses of Standard Preparation and the two doses of the preparation being examined should be given according to a randomized block or a Latin square design and at least six responses to each should be recorded.

Measure all the responses and calculate the result of the assay by standard statistical methods.

**Method C: By measurement of milk-ejection pressure in a lactating rat** — Select a lactating rat, in the third to twenty-first day after parturition and weighing about 300 g, separate it from the litter and 30 to 60 minutes later anaesthetise (for example, by the intraperitoneal injection of a solution of Pentobarbitone Sodium). Tie the rat to an operating table, maintained at 37°, by its hind legs leaving the front legs free. Cannulate the trachea with a short polyethylene tube of internal diameter about 2.5 mm in such a manner so as to ensure a free airway; apply artificial respiration only if necessary. Cannulate an external jugular or femoral vein with a polyethylene tube of internal diameter about 0.4 mm which is filled with saline solution and closed with a pin.

Shave the skin surrounding the inguinal and abdominal teats and excise the tip of one teat, preferably the lower inguinal teat. Insert a polyethylene tube of internal diameter about 0.3 mm and external diameter about 0.6 mm, to a depth sufficient to obtain appropriate measurement of pressure (3 to 10 mm depth), into the primary teat duct which opens onto the cut surface and tie firmly in place with a ligature. Connect this cannula with a suitable strain gauge transducer (such as that used for recording arterial blood pressure in the rat) and fill the whole system with a 3.8% w/v solution of sodium citrate or saline solution containing 50 Units of heparin sodium per ml to prevent clotting of milk. After cannulation, inject a small volume (0.05 to 0.2 ml) of this solution into the teat duct through the transducer to clear the milk from the tip of the cannula. (This procedure may be repeated during the assay should obstruction arise from milk ejected into the cannula). Clamp the strain gauge so that a slight tension is applied to the teat and its natural alignment is preserved and connect the gauge to a potentiometric recorder adjusted to give full-scale deflection for an increase in milk-ejection pressure of about 5.3 kPa. Inject all solutions through the venous cannula using a 1-ml syringe graduated in 0.01 ml and wash them in with 0.2 ml of saline solution.

Prepare a solution of the Standard Preparation and a solution of the preparation being examined in saline solution so that the volume to be injected is between 0.1 ml and 0.4 ml. Choose two doses of the Standard Preparation such that the increase in milk-ejection pressure is about 1.35 kPa for the lower dose and about 2.7 kPa for the higher dose. As an initial approximation, a lower dose of between 0.1 and 0.4 milliUnit and an upper dose of 1.5 to 2 times this amount may be tried. Choose two doses of the preparation being examined with the same inter-dose ratio, matching the effects of the doses of the Standard Preparation as closely as possible. Inject the four doses (two doses of the Standard Preparation and two doses of the preparation being examined) at intervals of 3 to 5 minutes. The two doses of Standard Preparation and the two doses of the preparation being examined should be given according to a randomised block or a Latin square design and at least four responses to each should be recorded. Measure all the responses and calculate the result of the assay by standard statistical methods.

## (viii). Biological Assay for Vasopressor Activity

**Principle:** The vasopressor activity is estimated by comparing the activity of the preparation being examined with that of the Standard Preparation of arginine vasopressin under the conditions of a suitable method of assay.

**Standard Preparation:** The Standard Preparation is the Ist International Standard for Arginine vasopressin, established in 1978, consisting of freeze-dried synthetic arginine vasopressin peptide acetate with human albumin and citric acid (supplied in ampoules containing 8.20 Units), or another suitable preparation the potency of which has been determined in relation to that of the International Standard.

**Suggested Method:** Inject slowly into the tail vein of a male albino rat weighing about 300 g a solution of a suitable alpha -adrenoceptor blocking agent, for example 10 ml per kg of body weight of a solution prepared by dissolving 5 mg of phenoxybenzamine hydrochloride in 0.1 ml of ethanol (95%), adding 0.05 ml of 1M hydrochloride acid and diluting to 5 ml with saline solution. After 18 hours, anaesthetise the rat with an anaesthetic that will maintain a prolonged and uniform blood pressure. After 45 to 60 minutes, tie the rat on its back to the operating table by its hind legs. Cannulate the trachea with a short polyethylene tube of external diameter about 2.5 mm and dissect a carotid artery ready for cannulation. Then cannulate the femoral vein close to the inguinal ligament. Retract the abdominal muscles to expose the inguinal ligament. Retract the superficial pudendal vein to one side and dissect the femoral vein towards the inguinal ligament from the corresponding artery. When dissecting, a deep branch reaching the femoral vein must be found and tied off to prevent bleeding during cannulation. Tie a short polyethylene cannula of external diameter about 1 mm into the femoral vein by two ligatures and join by a short piece of flexible tubing to a 1-ml burette with an attached thistle funnel containing saline solution at about 37°. Firmly fix a wet absorbent cotton swab to the thigh so as to cover the incision and cannula. At this stage inject through the venous cannula 200 Units of heparin, dissolved in saline solution, per 100 g of body weight. Then tie in a carotid cannula of external diameter about 1 mm and connect by a column of saline solution containing heparin with a suitable pressure measuring device such as a mercury manometer of internal diameter about 2 to 3 mm.

The central and peripheral nervous system including both vagus and associated sympathetic nerves is left intact. No artificial respiration is necessary. Taking care that no air is injected, inject all solutions through the venous cannula by means of a 1-ml syringe graduated in 0.01 ml and wash in with 0.2 ml of saline solution from the burette.

Dilute the extract of the Standard Preparation and the preparation being examined with saline solution so that the volume to be injected is between 0.1 ml and 0.5 ml. Choose two doses of the Standard Preparation such that the elevation of the blood pressure is about 4 kPa for the lower dose and about 7 kPa but always submaximal for the higher dose, the ratio of low to high dose being determined by the response and usually being 3 to 5. As an initial approximation doses of 3 and 5 milliUnits may be tried. Choose two doses of the preparation being examined with the same inter-dose ratio, matching the effects of the dose of the Standard Preparation as closely as possible. Inject doses at intervals of 10 to 15 minutes. The two doses of the Standard Preparation and the two doses of the preparation being examined should be given in a randomised block or a Latin square design and four to five responses to each should be recorded. Measure all the responses and calculate the result of the assay by standard statistical methods.

## (ix). Biological Assay of Chorionic Gonadotrophin

**Principle**: The potency of chorionic gonadotrophin is determined by comparing its effect in increasing the weight of the seminal vesicles or the prostate glands of immature rats with that of the Standard Preparation of chorionic gonadotrophin under the conditions of the following method of assay.

**Standard Preparation**: The Standard Preparation is the 3rd International Standard for Chorionic Gonadotrophin, human, established in 1986, consisting of a freeze-dried extract of human chorionic gonadotrophin with human albumin (supplied in ampoules containing 650 Units), or another suitable preparation the potency of which has been determined in relation to the International Standard.

**Suggested Method**: Use immature male rats of the same strain, approximately 21 days old and of approximately equal weight within the range 25 to 35 gm. Assign the rats at random to four equal groups of atleast eight animals. If sets of four litter mates are available, allot one litter mate from each set at random to each group and mark according to the litter.

Choose two doses of the Standard Preparation and two of the preparation being examined such that the smaller dose is sufficient to produce a positive response in some of the rats and the larger dose does not produce a maximum response in all of the rats. As an initial approximation, doses of 7.5 and 15 Units may be tried although the dose will depend on the sensitivity of the animals used which may vary widely. Dissolve separately the total quantities of the preparation being examined and of the Standard Preparation corresponding to the daily doses to be used in sufficient albumin-phosphate buffer pH 7.2 so that the daily dose is about 0.2 ml. Add a suitable antimicrobial preservative such as 0.4% w/v of phenol or 0.002% w/v of thiomersal. Store the solutions at a temperature of 2° to 8°. Inject subcutaneously into each rat the daily dose allocated to its group on 4 consecutive days at the same time each day. On the fifth day, about 24 hours after the last injection, kill the rats and remove the seminal vesicles or the prostate glands from each animal. Remove any extraneous fluid and tissue from the vesicles or glands and weigh them immediately. Calculate the result of the assay by standard statistical methods using the weight of the vesicles or prostate glands as the response.

## (x). Biological Assay of Urokinase

**Principle**: The potency of urokinase is determined by comparing its ability to activate human plasminogen to form plasmin with that of the Standard Preparation. The plasmin generated is determined by measurement of the time taken to lyse a fibrin clot under the conditions of a suitable method of assay.

**Standard Preparation:** The Standard Preparation is the 1st International Reference Preparation for Urokinase, human, established in 1968, consisting of partially purified freeze-dried urokinase from human urine with lactose (supplied in ampoules containing 4800 Units of urokinase activity) or another suitable preparation the activity of which has been determined in relation to the International Reference Preparation.

**Method**: Prepare a solution of the Standard Preparation containing 1000 Units of urokinase activity per ml and prepare a solution of the preparation being examined expected to have the same concentration; keep the solutions in ice and use within 6 hours. Prepare three 1.5-fold serial dilutions of the solution of the Standard Preparation so that the longest clot-lysis time is less than 20 minutes and the shortest clot-lysis time is greater than 3 minutes. Prepare three similar dilutions of the solution of the preparation being examined. Keep the solutions in ice and use within 1 hour. Using 24 tubes 8 mm in diameter, label the tubes $S_1$, $S_2$, $S_3$ for the dilutions of the Standard Preparation and $T_1$, $T_2$, $T_3$ for the dilutions of the preparation being examined, allocating four tubes to each dilution. Place the tubes in ice. Into each tube introduce 0.2 ml of the appropriate dilution, 0.2 ml of phosphate buffer pH 7.4 containing 3% w/v of bovine albumin and 0.1 ml of a solution containing 20 Units of thrombin per ml. Place the tubes in a water-bath at 37° and allow to stand for 2 minutes to attain temperature equilibrium. Using an automatic pipette, introduce into the bottom of the first tube 0.5 ml of a 1.0% w/v solution of bovine euglobulin fraction ensuring mixing. At 5-second intervals introduce successively into the remaining tubes 0.5 ml of a 1.0% w/v solution of bovine euglobulin fraction. Using a stop-watch, measure for each tube the time in seconds that elapses between the addition of the euglobulin and the lysis of the clot.

Using the logarithms of the lysis times, calculate the result of the assay by standard statistical methods.

## (xi). Biological Assay of Streptokinase

The potency of streptokinase is determined by comparing its ability to activate human plasminogen to form plasmin with that of the Standard Preparation. The plasmin generated is determined by measurement of the time taken to lyse a fibrin clot under the conditions of a suitable method of assay.

**Standard Preparation:** The Standard Preparation is the 2nd International Standard for Streptokinase, established in 1989, consisting of freeze-dried streptokinase (supplied in ampoules containing 700 Units of streptokinase activity), or another suitable preparation the activity of which has been determined in relation to the International reference preparation.

**Suggested Method :** Prepare a solution of the Standard Preparation to contain 1000 Units of streptokinase activity per ml and prepare a solution of the preparation being examined expected to have the same concentration; keep the solutions in ice and use within 6 hours. Prepare three 1.5-fold serial dilutions of the solution of the Standard Preparation so that the longest clot-lysis time is less than 20 minutes and prepare three similar dilutions of the solution of the preparation being examined. Keep the solutions in ice and use within 1 hour.

Using 24 tubes, 8 mm in diameter, label the tubes $S_1$, $S_2$, $S_3$ for the dilutions of the Standard Preparation and $T_1$, $T_2$, $T_3$ for the dilutions of the Standard Preparation being examined, allocating four tubes to each dilution. Place the tubes in ice. Into each tube introduce 0.2 ml of the appropriate dilution, 0.2 ml of citro-phosphate buffer pH 7.2 containing 3% w/v of bovine serum albumin and 0.1 ml of a solution containing 20 Units of thrombin per ml. Place the tubes in a water-bath at 37° and allow to stand for 2 minutes to attain temperature equilibrium. Using an automatic pipette, introduce into the bottom of the first tube 0.5 ml of a 1% w/v solution to human euglobulins ensuring mixing. At 5-second intervals introduce successively into the remaining tubes 0.5 ml of a 1% w/v solution of human euglobulins. Using a stop-watch, measure for each tube the time in seconds that elapses between the addition of the euglobulin and the lysis of the clot.

Using the logarithms of the lysis times, calculate the result of the assay by standard statistical methods.

## Current Status of Bioassay in Different Pharmacopoeia

The above mentioned bioassay have been routinely used in out of various bioassays mentioned above, some are used in academic institutions whereas official methods utilized in pharmaceutical industries. With the advent of technology, availability of advanced, sophisticated and more reliable analytical methods the scenario for bioassay has changed dramatically.

Pharmacopoeia, the official publication by competent government authorities of various countries, gives recommendations for analytical methods for various drugs to have assurance of quality of drugs. If one review the emphasis of bioassay in pharmacopeias published before 1980 as compared to those published recently, it will be clear that

(a) There are very few drugs which are now recommended to be assayed by biological methods.
(b) Most of the drugs which were assayed by biological methods are now being recommended to be assayed by chemical methods. (Table 2)
(c) Newer drugs have been included for which bioassay recommended.

**Table 2: List of drugs for which bioassay was recommended in earlier pharmacopoea,* now replaced by other methods:**

| S.No. | Names of Drugs | Assay method Recommended |
|---|---|---|
| 1. | Acetylcholine | Titrimetric method |
| 2. | Histamine | Titrimetric method |
| 3. | Heparin | Titrimetric method |
| 4. | Thyroxine | Titrimetric method |

| S.No. | Names of Drugs | Assay method Recommended |
|---|---|---|
| 5. | Adrenaline | UV absorbance |
| 6. | Progesterone | UV absorbance |
| 7. | Digoxin | UV absorbance |
| 8. | Estradiol | Chromatography |
| 9. | Penicillin | Chromatography |
| 10. | Insulin | HPLC |

In the Pharmacopea (USP-95, EP-97 and IP-96) oxytocin, heparin and chorionic gonadotrophins are included for bioassay. Corticotrophin and glucagen are also recommended to be assayed by biological method. In addition to these calcitonin, pancreatin and menotrophin are to be analyzed by bioassay according to BP 93 and Vitamin D, FSH and LH are to be bioassayed as per USP-95, IP-96 has included several vaccines, streptolkinase and prokinase in the list of bioassay

## Other Official Bioassays (As per Indian Pharmacopoeia 1996)

### 1. Biological Assay of Diphtheria Antitoxin

The potency of diphtheria antitoxin is determined by comparing the dose necessary to protect guinea-pigs or rabbits against the erythrogenic effects of a fixed dose of the Standard Preparation of diphtheria antitoxin necessary to give the same protection. For this purpose, a suitable preparation of diphtheria toxin is required to be used as a test toxin. The test dose of the toxin is determined in relation to the Standard Preparation. The potency of the preparation being examined is then determined in relation to the Standard Preparation using the test toxin.

**Standard Preparation:** The Standard Preparation is the Ist International Standard for Diphtheria antitoxin, equine, established in 1934, consisting of the dried hyperimmune horse serum and glycerin, or another suitable preparation the potency of which has been determined in relation to the International Standard.

#### Method:

**Test toxin**: Prepare diphtheria toxin by filtering through bacteria-proof filter the medium in which a toxigenic strain of C. diphtheriae has grown. Store at a temperature of 2° and 8°.

**Selection of test toxin**: In selecting a toxin for use as the test toxin determine the following:

Lr/100 dose — This is the smallest quantity of the toxin which, when mixed with 0.01 Unit of antitoxin and injected intracutaneously into guinea-pigs or rabbits causes a characteristic reaction at the site of the injection within 48 hours.

Minimal reacting dose — This is the smallest quantity of toxin which, when injected intracutaneously into guinea-pigs or rabbits, causes a characteristic reaction at the site of injection within 48 hours.

A suitable toxin is one which contains at least 200 minimal reacting doses in the Lr/100 dose. The test toxin is allowed to stand for some months before being used for the **assay** of samples of antitoxin. During this time its toxicity declines and the Lr/100 dose may be slightly increased. When experiment shows that the Lr/100 dose is constant, the test toxin is ready for use and may be used for a long period. Determine the minimal reacting dose and the Lr/100 dose at frequent intervals. Store the test toxin in the dark at a temperature between 0° and 5°. Maintain its sterility by the addition of toluene or other antimicrobial preservative which does not cause a rapid decline in specific toxicity.

**Determination of test dose of toxin** (Lr/100 dose): Prepare a solution of the Standard Preparation with saline solution such that 1 ml contains 0.1 Unit. Prepare mixtures such that 2.0 ml of each mixture contains 1.0 ml of the dilution of the Standard Preparation (0.1 Unit) and one of a series of graded volumes of the test toxin. Dilute each mixture with saline solution to the same final volume (2.0 ml). Allow the mixtures to stand at room temperature, protected from light, for 15 to 60 minutes and inject intracutaneously 0.2 ml of each mixture at suitably spaced sites into the shaven or depilated flanks of two animals. Observe the animals for 48 hours.

The test dose (Lr/100) of the toxin is the amount present in 0.2 ml of that mixture which causes at the site of injection a small, characteristic reaction in the skin of the guinea-pig or rabbit. Mixtures containing larger amounts of toxin cause larger reaction and necrosis and mixtures containing smaller amount of toxin cause no reaction.

**Determination of potency of the antitoxin**: Dilute the test toxin with saline solution so that 1.0 ml contains 10 times the test dose. Prepare mixtures such that 2.0 ml of each mixture contains 1.0 ml of the dilution of the toxin and one of a series of graded volumes of the preparation being examined. Prepare further mixtures such that 2.0 ml of each contains 1.0 ml of the solution of the test toxin and 0.1 Unit of antitoxin. Dilute each mixture with saline solution to the same final volume (2.0 ml). Allow the mixtures to stand at room temperature, protected from light, for 15 to 60 minutes. Inject a dose of 0.2 ml of each mixture into the animals under the conditions described in the determination of the Lr/100 dose of the toxin.

The mixture of the preparation being examined that contains 0.01 Unit of antitoxin in 0.2 ml is the mixture that produces the same degree of local reaction as that produced by the injection into the same animals of the mixture of the Standard Preparation that contains in 0.2 ml the test dose (Lr/100) of the toxin and 0.01 Unit of antitoxin.

When at least four distinct tests are carried out by this method, the limits of error have been estimated to be between 90% and 111%.

## 2. Biological Assay of Plague Vaccine

The potency of plague vaccine is estimated by determining the dose necessary to protect mice against a lethal dose of a virulent strain of Yersinia pestis.

**Test Animals**: Use white mice, 6 to 7 weeks old, each weighing between 20 and 28 g and of a strain susceptible to plague infection. The selected strain of mice should be such that an infective dose of 6 to 12 organisms of a virulent strain of Y. pestis per mouse given subcutaneously produces a mortality of not less than 80% of the animals used. The animals should be healthy and free from intercurrent infection with organisms such as Salmonella.

### Suggested Method:

**Selection of suitable virulent strain**: A freeze-dried virulent culture of Y. pestis, established to be suitable for challenge, is revived by sub-culturing 0.5 ml in 9.5 ml of nutrient broth contained in another test-tube and incubating at 28° for exactly 48 hours. Such a culture should contain 300 to 600 million organisms per ml. Make 10-fold dilutions in nutrient broth and test for virulence. Use a $10^{-7}$ dilution containing 6 to 12 organisms in 0.2 ml as the test infective dose per animal. Those strains which produce a mortality of 80% among the animals tested with this dose are considered to be virulent.

**Standard challenge dose**: Freshly reconstitute the freeze-dried culture and dilute with nutrient broth to a strength such that 0.2 ml contains 60 to 120 organisms.

**Measurement of protective power**: Prepare a series of five graded doses of the preparation being examined arranged in such a manner that the 50% protective dose ($ED_{50}$) lies about the middle of the selected series. For each dose a batch of 16 mice is used. Inject subcutaneously the selected dose in two equal parts with an interval of 7 days between them. Seven days after the second half of the dose, inject subcutaneously into each group of mice the standard challenge dose. At the same time inject into 10 control mice, 8 to 9 weeks old and weighing between 28 g and 30 g, the standard challenge dose.

Observe the animals for 15 days and record the number of deaths in each group. Carry out a post-mortem on the dead animals and look for signs of plague in them. If plague organisms are not seen, such deaths are excluded from the calculation. The test is not valid unless the number of such deaths is not more than 1. At the end of the period of observation kill all the surviving animals and examine for signs of plague. Calculate the median effective immunizing dose, $ED_{50}$, by standard statistical methods. The vaccine passes the test if it has an $ED_{50}$ of 0.004 ml or less per mouse.

# VIVA-VOCE

**Q.1 Define bioassay.**

**Ans:** Bioassay may be defined as the determination of the concentration of a biologically active substance, of physical, chemical or biological origin, by using a biological indicator with reference to standard.

**Q.2 Write the applications of bioassay.**

**Ans:**

1. To standardize drugs of natural origin, especially when the chemical identity of the active has not been elucidated fully. e.g: parathyroid hormones, antitoxins etc.
2. To standardize those drugs from which no adequate chemical assay has been devised even though the chemical structure of the active principle has been established.e.g: Hormones like insulin, oxytocin etc.
3. To standardize the drugs which are composed of a complex mixture of substances varying structure and activity. e.g: digitalis, posterior pituitary extract etc.
4. If the chemical assay is not a valid indication of the biological activity, e.g. due to lack of differentiation between active and inactive isomers.
5. To standardize when the drugs have same pharmacological actions but different chemical structures existing together. e.: glycosides in digitalis preparation.
6. To estimate the dose of a drug required to produce a therapeutic or toxic response. e.g: calculation of ED50, LD50 etc.
7. When the physical property of rotation (dextro or levo) shows difference in action. e.g: d- Chloramphenicol is active. Levo adrenaline is 80 times more active than dextro.

**Q.3 Write down the types of bioassay.**

**Ans:** 1. Quantal bioassay 2. Graded bioassay (Interpolation, Matching, Bracketing, multiple point bioassay)

**Q.4 Write down the principles of bioassay.**

**Ans:** The basic principle of bioassay is to compare the test substance with the international standard preparation of the same and to find out how much test substance is required to produce the same biological effect, as produced by the standard. The followings are the principles of bioassay:

1. All bioassays (lab studies, toxicity studies, clinical studies) must be comparative & compared against a standard drug or preparation. The potency of biologically assayed compounds is compared with the activity of internationally accepted standards.

2. The standard and new drugs should be as far as possible identical to each other, then their dose response curve (DRC) will have the same stop and would be constant all along the response level.
3. The biological response should be closely related to the therapeutic use of the drug as possible. For example, in estimating the potency of insulin, blood glucose levels would be of the ideal index, but the method commonly used is the mouse convulsion method, in which the % of animals developing convulsions are recorded. Similarly for estimating digitaloid drug, the arrest of heart in pigeon or guinea pig is used as end point which is as the toxic effect of the drug and not the therapeutic effect.
4. An estimate of relative potency is made by comparing the log dose of the test and the log dose of the standard that produces an equal magnitude of effect.
5. The problem of biological variation must be minimized as far as possible. For that one should keep uniform experimental conditions and assure the reproducibility of the responses. The results of the test should be subjected to statistical analysis to minimize errors due to biological variations.

**Q.5 Write down the advantages of bioassay.**

**Ans: Advantages:**

1. A chemical assay finds out only the amount of active substance present in a given sample where as the bioassay measures the actual biological activity of the active substance.
2. Bioassay measures small traces of compound too.
3. Bioassay can establish the biological activity of a substance even when its chemical identity is not known.
4. Sensitivity of a bioassay is greater than a chemical assay.
5. Chemical unstable drugs can be conveniently assayed by a bioassay.
6. The active and the inactive isomers present in a racemic mixture can be easily distinguished by a bioassay.

**Q.6 Write down the disadvantages of bioassay.**

**Ans: Disadvantages:**

1. Complicated set up.
2. Expensive.
3. Time consuming.
4. Too laborious
5. Requires skilled labor.
6. The effect observed in animals may not be observed in humans.
7. The quantitative accuracy of a bioassay usually falls considerably below that attainable with most chemical assays.

# Experiment No. 9

## Object: To perform bioassay of Acetylcholine by matching method on Guinea pig ileum preparation.

## Principle:

It is the most simple type of bioassay. In this type of bioassay the response of the test substance is taken first and the observed response is tried to match with the response that is obtained with the standard drugs. Several responses of standard drug are recorded till a close matching response to that of test substance is observed. A corresponding concentration is thus calculated. This assay is employed when the sample size is very small. Since the assay does not involve the recording of concentration response curve, the sensitivity of the preparation is not taken into consideration. Therefore, the precision and reliability are not very good by this method.

In this, the dose of test is constant where as standard dose is vary. The given formula of matching method as mentioned below:

$$\text{Concentration of unknown} = \frac{\text{Dose of standard}}{\text{Dose of test}} \times \text{Concentration of Standard}$$

## Requirements:

**Animal:** Guinea pig (400-600 gm)

**Drugs:** Acetylcholine

**Physiological solution:** Tyrode

**Apparatus:** Student's single unit organ bath, aeration or oxygen delivery tube, isotonic frontal writing lever, fulcrum, Sherrington's recording drum, reservoir etc.

## Experimental conditions:

Temperature: 30-32°C

Tension of lever: 0.5gm

Magnification: 10 times

Aeration: 70-72 bubble/min

## Procedure:

1. The assembly is set up and arrangements are made for experimental conditions mentioned above.
2. Guinea pig which is fasted overnight sacrificed as per CPCSEA recommended guidelines.
3. The abdominal cavity is quickly opened and a piece of ileum is isolated.
4. It placed in a petri dish containing tyrode solution maintaining at 32°C.
5. Mount the preparation in up-right position in the organ bath containing tyrode solution under a tension of 0.5 g.
6. Relax the tissue for 45 min, during which period wash the tissue with fresh quantum of tyrode for at least four times.
7. Record the concentrations due to acetylcholine using frontal writing lever. 90 second contact time and a total 5 min time cycle may be used for proper recording of the responses.
8. Concentration dependent responses due to Ach and test solution were recorded using frontal writing lever.
9. From DRC, two doses of the standard and one dose of the test solution were chosen which lies in the linear part of the curve.
10. The extent of contraction produced by the test sample is compared with standard preparation of acetylcholine.
11. The response of the standard, which matches, with that of the unknown sample would be found by trial and error method.
12. The response of the standard, which matches, with that of the unknown is matched.
13. Graph is fixed using fixing solution and the potency of the sample is determined and expressed as µg/ml.

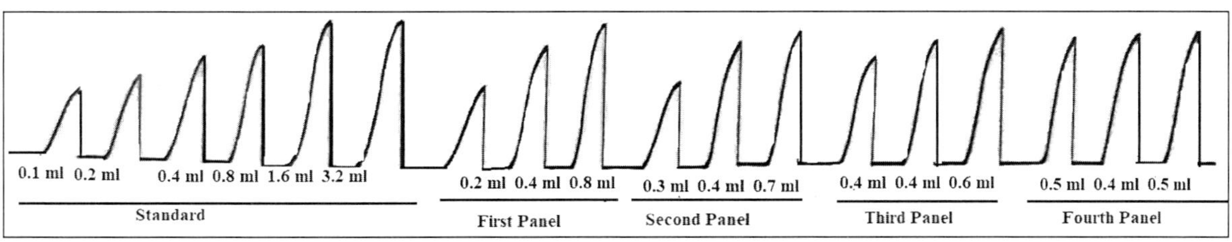


**Bioassay of Acetylcholine by matching method**

## Precaution:

1. As per dilution concentration of drug is prepared.
2. DRC taken as per manner.
3. Use thin piece (2-3cm) as it is more sensitive than bulky piece.
4. The level of PSS in the organ bath should remain constant throughout the experiment by marking the level with elastic ring/marker.
5. Speed of the drum should be slow (0.25mm) and the lever should be placed tangential to the drum.
6. The no. of washing and the interval between them should be kept constant.
7. Organ bath containing tyrode solution maintained at 30-32°C

## VIVA-VOCE

**Q.1 Define matching bioassay.**

**Ans:** In this type of bioassay the response of the test substance is taken first and the observed response is tried to match with the response that is obtained with the standard drugs. Several responses of standard drug are recorded till a close matching response to that of test substance is observed.

**Q.2 How to prepare isolated guinea pig ileum tissue.**

**Ans:** Abdominal wall is dissected out so as to isolate the ileum, the faecal matter, mesentery and blood vessels are removed from the piece of ileum. It is ligated on both sides and suspended in mammalian organ bath containing tyrode solution maintained 30-32°C and oxygenated continuously.

**Q.3 Write down the formula of matching method.**

**Ans:**

$$\text{Concentration of unknown} = \frac{\text{Dose of standard}}{\text{Dose of test}} \times \text{Concentration of Standard}$$

# Experiment No. 10

## Object: To perform bioassay of oxytocin using rat uterus preparations by interpolation method.

## Principle:

Interpolation method of bioassay is less time consuming and yet reliable as compared to matching type of bioassay. One of the main advantages of this assay is that the sensitivity of the tissue is first determined by prior plotting of a concentration-response curve with the known agonist. If the linearity of the curve is good, one can do very accurate estimate of the test substance.

This method is based on the assumption of dose-response relationship. Log dose response curve is plotted and the dose of the standard producing the same response as produced by the test sample is directly read from the graph so as to estimate the potency of the test sample. This is a simplest form of graded response assay and involves no statistical data and many calculations. In this assay the dose response curve is first obtained from different doses of standard solution. The concentration of unknown is then read from the standard graph.

Oxytocin is a hormone secreted by the posterior pituitary gland. The rat uterine preparation is commonly used for the bioassay of oxytocin. The sensitivity of the uterus to oxytocin depends on the oestrous cycle. The various stages of oestrous cycle can be identified by preparing vaginal smears and observing under microscope. Rat uterus is highly sensitive.

## Requirements:

**Animal:** Female rat (120-150 g)

**Drugs:** Oxytocin, Stilbestrol

**Physiological solution:** De jalon

**Apparatus:** Student's single unit organ bath, aeration or oxygen delivery tube, isotonic frontal writing lever, fulcrum, Sherrington's recording drum, reservoir, pinch cork, screw clip etc.

## Experimental conditions:

Temperature: 30-32°C

Tension of lever: 0.5gm

Magnification: 10 times

Aeration: 70-72 bubble/min

## Procedure:

### A. preparation of animal:

1. Examine the vaginal smear under microscope to know about the proper stage of oestrus cycle. If the rat is not in frank oestrus, inject 0.1 mg/kg of stilbestrol and wait for 24 hr. (Vaginal smear is prepared by taking a drop of vaginal wash and putting on the glass slide).
2. If the epithelial cells are present in the smear, it is said to be in frank oestrous phase.

### B. Isolation of tissue:

1. Animal is sacrificed by cervical dislocation.
2. Cut open the pelvic region and expose both the horns of uterus. Separate them gently from the surrounding fatty material and transfer them into a dish containing De jalon's solution. When the rat is in oestrus stage the uterus is fleshy and pink in colour due to increased vascularity.
3. Then the uterus is cut longitudinally and a tissue portion of 2-3 cm long is taken and both ends are tied with the thread.
4. One end of the tissue is tied to the aeration tube cum tissue holder and the other end is tied to the isotonic frontal writing lever.

### C. Mounting the tissue:

1. About 2-3 cm long tissue is mounted in organ bath containing De jalons solution along with proper aeration.
2. A tension of about 500 mg (0.5g) is applied and tissue is allowed to equilibrate for 45 min.

### D. Recording of the response:

1. Record the DRC for the standard oxytocin solution is taken.
2. A contact time of 30 sec and 3 minutes time cycle is used for proper recording of the responses.

3. Record responses due to 0.1, 0.2, or 0.4 ml of the test substance. See that these responses would fall on the linear portion of the concentration –response curve for the stand solution
4. Label and fix the tracing.
5. Plot the graph with log dose on X-axis and % response on Y-axis and interpolate the test response on the DRC of standard.
6. Calculate the potency of the test drug by converting the log of the standard dose that has produced an equivalent response as that of test in to anti-log and report the potency as number of μg/ml.

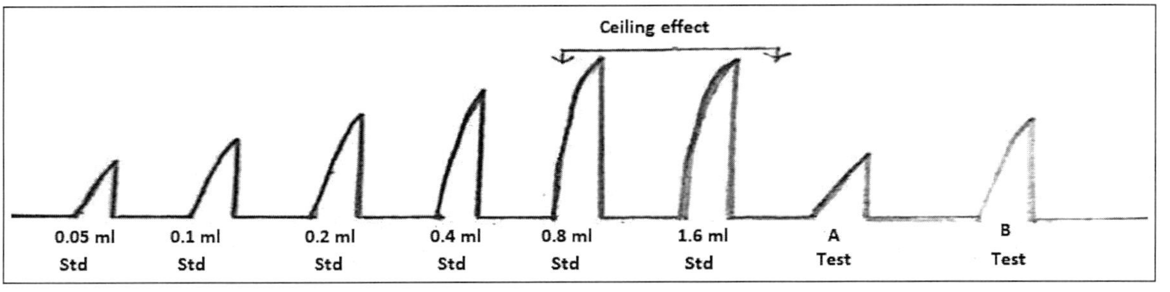


**Bioassay of oxytocin by interpolation method.**

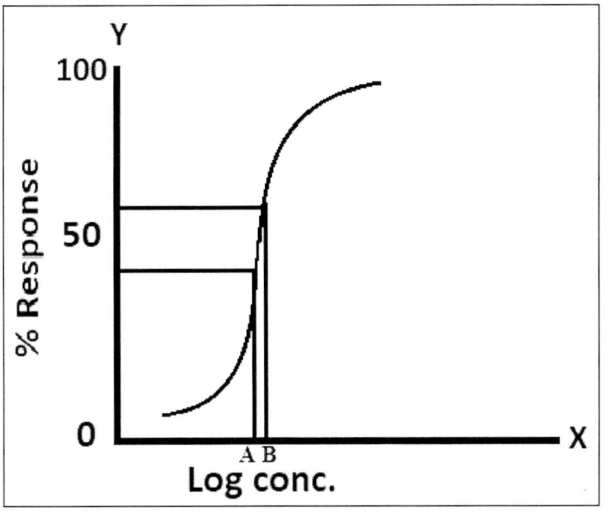


**Concentration response curves**

## Observation Table:

| Standard Solution | | | | | | |
|---|---|---|---|---|---|---|
| S.No. | Conc. of std. soltution (µg/ml) | Dose of std. solution (ml) | Concentration in (µg) | Log concentration | Response height (mm) | % Response height |
| 1. | | 0.05 | 50 | 1.698 | | |
| 2. | | 0.1 | 100 | 2 | | |
| 3. | | 0.2 | 200 | 2.301 | | |
| 4. | | 0.4 | 400 | 2.602 | | |
| 5. | | 0.8 | 800 | 2.903 | | |
| 6. | | 1.6 | 1600 | 3.204 | | |
| **Test Solution** | | | | | | |
| **S.No.** | **Conc. of test soltution (µg/ml)** | **Dose of test (ml)** | **Concentration (µg)** | **Log concentration** | **Response height (mm)** | **% Response height** |
| 1. | - | 0.1 | 100 | 2 | | |
| 2. | - | 0.2 | 200 | 2.301 | | |

## Precautions:

1. Cut out all the blood capillaries present on muscle preparation by using a sharp scissor.
2. Use thin piece (2-3cm) as it is more sensitive than bulky piece.
3. The level of PSS in the organ bath should remain constant throughout the experiment by marking the level with elastic ring/marker.
4. Speed of the drum should be slow (0.25mm) and the lever should be placed tangential to the drum.
5. The no. of washing and the interval between them should be kept constant.
6. Carefully mounting of the uterine preparation.
7. Organ bath containing De jalone solution maintained at 30-32°C
8. Examine the vaginal smear under microscope

# VIVA-VOCE

**Q.1 What do you mean by interpolation.**

**Ans:** This method is based on the assumption of dose-response relationship. Log dose response curve is plotted and the dose of the standard producing the same response as produced by the test sample is directly read from the graph so as to estimate the potency of the test sample. This is a simplest form of graded response assay and involves no statistical data and many calculations. In this assay the dose response curve is first obtained from different doses of standard solution. The concentration of unknown is then read from the standard graph.

**Q.2 Why we apply additional weight on the long arm of lever.**

**Ans:** Because of trauma during dissection, the muscle goes into a state of spasm. Additional weight of (0.5-1 gm) is applied so that, the muscle relaxed properly and regain its original length so better contractile responses are recorded.

**Q.3 Write down the full form of DRC.**

**Ans:** The form of DRC is Dose Response Concentration.

# Experiment No. 11

## Object: To perform bioassay of oxytocin using rat uterus preparations by three point method.

## Principle:

It is a method based on the assumption of dose-response relationship. Log dose response curve is plotted and the dose of the standard producing the same response as produced by the test sample is directly read from the graph so to estimate the potency of the test sample.

In three point bioassay, the DRC of standard, test samples is first obtained from the responses due to graded doses. From the DRC of standard, two standard doses are selected in such a way that they have produced 25% and 75% of the maximal response respectively and are designated as S1 and S2. The responses of these doses lie on the steepest and straightest part (linear) of the curve. From The DRC of test sample one test dose is selected such that it gives a response which lies in between the two standard responses i.e. it gives a greater response than S1 and a smaller response than S2 and is designated as T.

After selecting the standard and test doses, the bioassay is performed by recording the standard and test responses in a randomized fashion. The pattern of addition of doses is S1, S2, T; S2, T, S1 and T, S1, S2 in 3 successive cycles. The mean values of height of the contraction for all the 3 doses are calculated and are used in plotting the graph so as to estimate the potency of the test sample.

Oxytocin is a hormone secreted by the posterior pituitary gland. The rat uterine preparation is commonly used for the bioassay of oxytocin. The sensitivity of the uterus to oxytocin depends on the oestrous cycle. The various stages of oestrous cycle can be identified by preparing vaginal smears and observing under microscope. Rat uterus is highly sensitive.

## Requirements:

**Animal:** Female rat (120-150 g)

**Drugs:** Oxytocin

**Physiological solution:** De jalon

**Apparatus:** Student's single unit organ bath, aeration or oxygen delivery tube, isotonic frontal writing lever, fulcrum, Sherrington's recording drum, reservoir, pinch cork, screw clip etc.

## Experimental conditions:

Temperature: 30-32°C

Tension of lever: 0.5gm

Magnification: 10 times

Aeration: 70-72 bubble/min

## Procedure:

### A. preparation of animal:

1. Examine the vaginal smear under microscope to know about the proper stage of oestrus cycle. If the rat is not in frank oestrus, inject 0.1 mg/kg of stilbestrol and wait for 24 hr.(Vaginal smear is prepared by taking a drop of vaginal wash and putting on the glass slide).
2. If the epithelial cells are present in the smear, it is said to be in frank oestrous phase.

### B. Isolation of tissue:

1. Animal is sacrificied by cervical dislocation.
2. Cut open the pelvic region and expose both the horns of uterus. Separate them gently from the surrounding fatty material and transfer them into a dish containing De jalon's solution. When the rat is in oestrus stage the uterus is fleshy and pink in colour due to increased vascularity.
3. Then the uterus is cut longitudinally and a tissue portion of 2-3 cm long is taken and both ends are tied with the thread.
4. One end of the tissue is tied to the aeration tube cum tissue holder and the other end is tied to the isotonic frontal writing lever.

### C. Mounting the tissue:

1. About 2-3 cm long tissue is mounted in organ bath containing De jalons solution along with proper aeration.
2. A tension of about 500 mg (0.5g) is applied and tissue is allowed to equilibrate for 45 min.

## D. Recording of the response:

1. Record the DRC for the standard oxytocin solution is taken.
2. A contact time of 90 sec and 5 minutes time cycle is used for proper recording of the responses.
3. Select two doses from DRC of standard drug, two standard doses are selected in such a way that they have produced 25% and 75 % of the maximal response respectively and are designated as S1 and S2.
4. Similarly, record the concentrations due to graded doses of test oxytocin. Select one dose from the DRC of test solution in such a way that the response due to this dose lies preferentially between $S_1$ and $S_2$ and designate it as T.
5. Record 3 sets of responses due to S1 S2 and T adding them to organ bath in a randomized fashion as per Latin square design mentioned in the princilple.The latin square design of addition of doses is followed to ensure good randomization and to account for the fluctuating sensitivity of the tissue.
6. Measure various response to calculate the mean of each response(S1,S2,T)
7. Plot the graph with log dose on X-Axis and % of response on Y –axis and interpolate the T response on to the DRC of standard in between S1 and S2 so as to find the standard dose that gives an equivalent response of that of test.
8. Calculate the potency of the test drug by converting the log of the standard dose that has produced an equivalent response as that of test in to anti-log and report the potency as number of µg/ml.
9. The concentration of test can also be determined mathematically with the help of the following formula:

**Concentration of unknown = $n_1/t \times \text{anti log} \{T\text{-}S_1 / S_{2\text{-}}S_1 \times \log n_2/n_1\}$ Cs**

n1 = Lower Standard dose
n2 = Higher Standard dose
t = Test dose
S1 = Response of n1
S2 = Response of n2
T = Response of test (t)
Cs = Concentration of standard

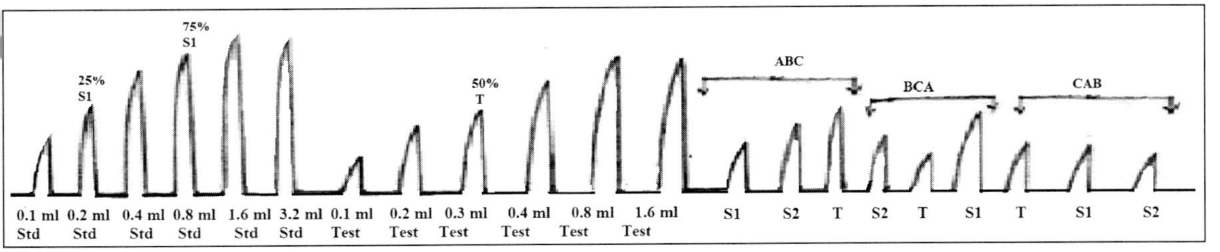


**Bioassay of oxytocin by using three point method.**

## Observation table:

| S.No. | Conc. of std. (μg/ml) | Type of Dose | Dose (ml) | Response height (mm) |
|---|---|---|---|---|
| 1. | | Standard | 0.1 | |
| 2. | | Standard | 0.2 ($S_1$) | |
| 3. | | Standard | 0.4 | |
| 4. | | Standard | 0.8 ($S_2$) | |
| 5. | | Standard | 1.6 | |
| 6. | | Standard | 3.2 | |
| 7. | | Test | 0.1 | |
| 8. | | Test | 0.2 | |
| 9. | | Test | 0.4 (T) | |
| 10. | | Test | 0.8 | |
| 11. | | Test | 1.6 | |
| 12. | | Test | 3.2 | |
| 13. | | $S_1$ | 0.2 | |
| 14. | | $S_2$ | 0.8 | |
| 15. | | T | 0.4 | |
| 16. | | $S_2$ | 0.8 | |
| 17. | | T | 0.4 | |
| 18. | | $S_1$ | 0.2 | |
| 19. | | T | 0.4 | |
| 20. | | $S_1$ | 0.2 | |
| 21. | | $S_2$ | 0.8 | |

## Precautions:

1. Cut out all the blood capillaries present on muscle preparation by using a sharp scissor.
2. Use thin piece (2-3cm) as it is more sensitive than bulky piece.
3. The level of PSS in the organ bath should remain constant throughout the experiment by marking the level with elastic ring/marker.
4. Speed of the drum should be slow (0.25mm) and the lever should be placed tangential to the drum.
5. The no. of washing and the interval between them should be kept constant.
6. Carefully mounting of the uterine preparation.
7. Organ bath containing De jalone solution maintained at 30-32°C
8. Examine the vaginal smear under microscope

## VIVA-VOCE

**Q.1 What is mean by three point bioassay.**

**Ans:** It is a method based on the assumption of dose-response relationship. Log dose response curve is plotted and the dose of the standard producing the same response as produced by the test sample is directly read from the graph so to estimate the potency of the test sample.

**Q.2 Which pattern is given in responses.**

**Ans:** The pattern of addition of doses is S1, S2, T; S2, T, S1 and T, S1, S2 in 3 successive cycles.

**Q.3 Give the formula of three point bioassay.**

**Ans:** Concentration of unknown = $n_1/t \times$ anti log $\{T\text{-}S_1 / S_{2\text{-}}S_1 \times \log n_2/n_1\}$ Cs

# Experiment No. 12

## Object: Bioassay of acetylcholine using guinea pig ileum by four point method.

## Principle:

This method is almost similar to the three point bioassay, but in this method 2 doses of the standard and the 2 doses of the test are used. The section of the standard doses should be such that they lie on the linear portion of the CRC and also the ratio between the smaller to greater dose should be preferably 1:2. The selection of the test doses is done by hit and trial method so that the responses fall on the linear part of the curve. By employing the latin square design, the responses of the chosen standard and the test doses is recorded in 4 successive cycles, in the order of

- $S_1, S_2, T_1, T_2$
- $S_2, T_1, T_2, S_1$
- $T_1, T_2, S_1, S_2$
- $T_2, S_1, S_2, T_1$

Guinea pig ileum is a smooth muscle preparation, used for assay of various drugs. Guinea pig ileum is also of choice for the assay due to its less spontaneous activity when compared to rabbit intestinal preparation. Once the tissue is mounted, when the spontaneous movements of the muscle subside, the effect of drug added to the bath is studied. If the test drug causes a contraction, it is a stimulant to smooth muscle.

## Requirements:

**Animal:** Guinea pig (400-600 g)

**Drugs:** Acetylcholine

**Physiological solution:** Tyrode

**Apparatus:** Student's single unit organ bath, aeration or oxygen delivery tube, isotonic frontal writing lever, fulcrum, Sherrington's recording drum, reservoir, pinch cork, screw clip etc.

## Experimental conditions:

Temperature: 30-32°C

Tension of lever: 0.5gm

Magnification: 10 times

Aeration: 70-72 bubble/min

## Procedure:

1. The assembly is set up and arrangements are made for experimental conditions mentioned above.
2. Guinea pig which is fasted overnight sacrificed as per CPCSEA recommended guidelines.
3. The abdominal cavity is quickly opened and a piece of ileum is isolated.
4. It placed in a petri dish containing tyrode solution maintaining at 32°C.
5. Mount the preparation in up-right position in the organ bath containing tyrode solution under a tension of 0.5 g.
6. Relax the tissue for 45 min, during which period wash the tissue with fresh quantum of tyrode for at least four times.
7. Record the concentrations due to acetylcholine using frontal writing lever. 90 second contact time and a total 5 min time cycle may be used for proper recording of the responses.
8. Concentration dependent responses due to Ach and test solution were recorded using frontal writing lever.
9. From DRC, two doses of the standard and two doses of the test solution were chosen which lies in the linear part of the curve.
10. They were named as $S_1$, S2, $T_1$ and $T_2$, where the response of $S_2$ should be double than the response of $S_{1.}$
11. The response of $T_1$ (dose) should lie in between $S_1$ and $S_{2.}$ $T_2$ (dose) should be double than that of $T_{1.}$
12. Their ratios $S_{1:}$ $S_2$ and $T_{1:}$ $T_2$ were preferably equal ($S_1 < T_1 < S_2 < T_2$)
13. Four sets of responses were recorded by adding them to the organ bath in a randomized fashion-latin square design as follows.

| | | | |
|---|---|---|---|
| $S_1$ | $S_2$ | $T_1$ | $T_2$ |
| $S_2$ | $T_1$ | $T_2$ | $S_1$ |
| $T_1$ | $T_2$ | $S_1$ | $S_2$ |
| $T_2$ | $S_1$ | $S_2$ | $T_1$ |

The potency ratio was calculated using following formula:

**Concentration of unknown = $n_1/t_1 \times$ anti log $\{(S_1+S_2)-(T_1+T_2)/(S_2+T_2)-(S_1+T_1)\times \log n_2/n_1\}$ Cs**

n1 = Lower Standard dose
n2 = Higher Standard dose
$t_1$ = Lower Test dose
$t_2$= Higher test dose
S1 = Mean of response of std ($S_1$)
S2 = Mean of response of std ($S_2$)
$T_1$ = Mean of response of test ($t_1$)
$T_2$ = Mean response of test ($t_2$)

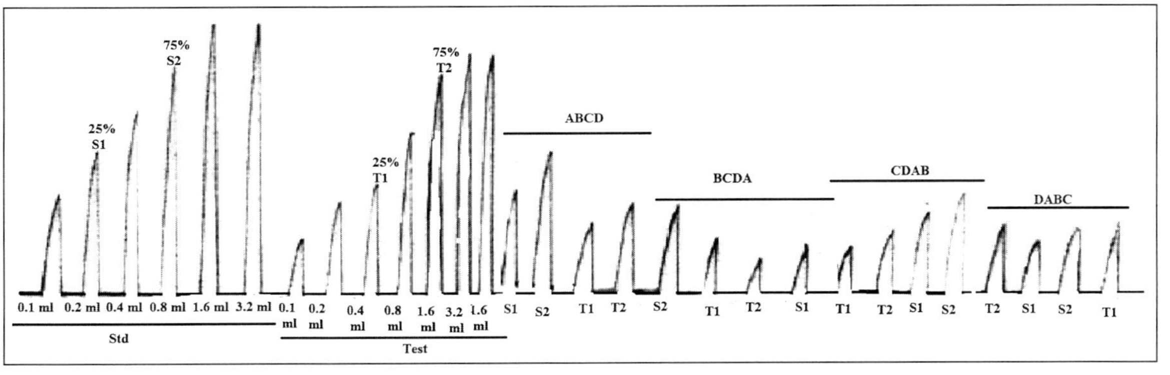


**Bioassay of acetylcholine by using four point method.**

## Observation table:

| S.No. | Conc. of std. (µg/ml) | Type of Dose | Dose (ml) | Response height (mm) |
|---|---|---|---|---|
| 1. | | Standard | 0.1 | |
| 2. | | Standard | 0.2 ($S_1$) | |
| 3. | | Standard | 0.4 | |
| 4. | | Standard | 0.8 ($S_2$) | |
| 5. | | Standard | 1.6 | |
| 6. | | Standard | 3.2 | |
| 7. | | Test | 0.1 | |
| 8. | | Test | 0.2 | |
| 9. | | Test | 0.4 ($T_1$) | |

| S.No. | Conc. of std. (μg/ml) | Type of Dose | Dose (ml) | Response height (mm) |
|---|---|---|---|---|
| 10. | | Test | 0.8 | |
| 11. | | Test | 1.6 ($T_2$) | |
| 12. | | Test | 3.2 | |
| 13. | | Test | 6.4 | |
| 14. | | $S_1$ | 0.2 | |
| 15. | | $S_2$ | 0.8 | |
| 16. | | $T_1$ | 0.4 | |
| 17. | | $T_2$ | 1.6 | |
| 18. | | $S_2$ | 0.8 | |
| 19. | | $T_1$ | 0.4 | |
| 20. | | $T_2$ | 1.6 | |
| 21. | | $S_1$ | 0.2 | |
| 22. | | $T_1$ | 0.4 | |
| 23. | | $T_2$ | 1.6 | |
| 24. | | $S_1$ | 0.2 | |
| 25. | | $S_2$ | 0.8 | |
| 26. | | $T_2$ | 1.6 | |
| 27. | | $S_1$ | 0.2 | |
| 28. | | $S_2$ | 0.8 | |
| 29. | | $T_1$ | 0.4 | |

## Precautions:

1. Cut out all the blood capillaries present on muscle preparation by using a sharp scissor.
2. Use thin piece (2-3cm) as it is more sensitive than bulky piece.
3. The level of PSS in the organ bath should remain constant throughout the experiment by marking the level with elastic ring/marker.
4. Speed of the drum should be slow (0.25mm) and the lever should be placed tangential to the drum.
5. The no. of washing and the interval between them should be kept constant.
6. Carefully mounting of the ileum preparation.
7. Organ bath containing tyrode solution maintained at 30-32°C

# VIVA-VOCE

**Q.1 What is mean by four point bioassay.**

**Ans:** This method is almost similar to the three point bioassay, but in this method 2 doses of the standard and the 2 doses of the test are used. The section of the standard doses should be such that they lie on the linear portion of the CRC and also the ratio between the smaller to greater dose should be preferably 1:2. The selection of the test doses is done by hit and trial method so that the responses fall on the linear part of the curve.

**Q.2 Which pattern is given in responses.**

**Ans:** The pattern of doses is

| | | | |
|---|---|---|---|
| $S_1$ | $S_2$ | $T_1$ | $T_2$ |
| $S_2$ | $T_1$ | $T_2$ | $S_1$ |
| $T_1$ | $T_2$ | $S_1$ | $S_2$ |
| $T_2$ | $S_1$ | $S_2$ | $T_1$ |

**Q.3 Give the formula of four point bioassay.**

**Ans:**

Concentration of unknown = $n_1/t_1 \times$ anti log $\{(S_1+S_2)-(T_1+T_2)/(S_2+T_2)-(S_1+T_1)\times \log n_2/n_1\}$ Cs

# Experiment No. 13

## Object: Bioassay of oxytocin using rat uterus preparation by four point method.

## Principle:

This method is almost similar to the three point bioassay, but in this method 2 doses of the standard and the 2 doses of the test are used. The section of the standard doses should be such that they lie on the linear portion of the CRC and also the ratio between the smaller to greater dose should be preferably 1:2. The selection of the test doses is done by hit and trial method so that the responses fall on the linear part of the curve. By employing the latin square design, the responses of the chosen standard and the test doses is recorded in 4 successive cycles, in the order of

- $S_1, S_2, T_1, T_2$
- $S_2, T_1, T_2, S_1$
- $T_1, T_2, S_1, S_2$
- $T_2, S_1, S_2, T_1$

Oxytocin is a hormone secreted by the posterior pituitary gland. The rat uterine preparation is commonly used for the bioassay of oxytocin. The sensitivity of the uterus to oxytocin depends on the oestrous cycle. The various stages of oestrous cycle can be identified by preparing vaginal smears and observing under microscope. Rat uterus is highly sensitive.

## Requirements:

**Animal:** Female rat (120-150 g)

**Drugs:** Oxytocin

**Physiological solution:** De jalon

**Apparatus:** Student's single unit organ bath, aeration or oxygen delivery tube, isotonic frontal writing lever, fulcrum, Sherrington's recording drum, reservoir, pinch cork, screw clip etc.

## Experimental conditions:

Temperature: 30-32°C

Tension of lever: 0.5gm

Magnification: 10 times

Aeration: 70-72 bubble/min

## Procedure:

### A. preparation of animal:

1. Examine the vaginal smear under microscope to know about the proper stage of oestrus cycle. If the rat is not in frank oestrus, inject 0.1 mg/kg of stilbestrol and wait for 24 hr (Vaginal smear is prepared by taking a drop of vaginal wash and putting on the glass slide).
2. If the epithelial cells are present in the smear, it is said to be in frank oestrous phase.

### B. Isolation of tissue:

1. Animal is sacrificied by cervical dislocation.
2. Cut open the pelvic region and expose both the horns of uterus. Separate them gently from the surrounding fatty material and transfer them into a dish containing De jalon's solution. When the rat is in oestrus stage the uterus is fleshy and pink in colour due to increased vascularity.
3. Then the uterus is cut longitudinally and a tissue portion of 2-3 cm long is taken and both ends are tied with the thread.
4. One end of the tissue is tied to the aeration tube cum tissue holder and the other end is tied to the isotonic frontal writing lever.

### C. Mounting the tissue:

1. About 2-3 cm long tissue is mounted in organ bath containing De jalons solution along with proper aeration.
2. A tension of about 500 mg (0.5g) is applied and tissue is allowed to equilibrate for 45 min.

### D. Recording of the response:

1. Record the DRC for the standard oxytocin solution is taken.
2. Record the concentrations due to oxytocin using frontal writing lever. 90 second contact time and a total 5 min time cycle may be used for proper recording of the responses.
3. Concentration dependent responses due to oxytocin and test solution were recorded using frontal writing lever.

4. From DRC, two doses of the standard and two doses of the test solution were chosen which lies in the linear part of the curve.
5. They were named as $S_1$, S2, $T_1$ and $T_2$, where the response of $S_2$ should be double than the response of $S_1$.
6. The response of $T_1$ (dose) should lie in between $S_1$ and $S_2$. $T_2$ (dose) should be double than that of $T_1$.
7. Their ratios $S_1$: $S_2$ and $T_1$: $T_2$ were preferably equal ($S_1 < T_1 < S_2 < T_2$)
8. Four sets of responses were recorded by adding them to the organ bath in a randomized fashion-latin square design as follows.

| | | | |
|---|---|---|---|
| $S_1$ | $S_2$ | $T_1$ | $T_2$ |
| $S_2$ | $T_1$ | $T_2$ | $S_1$ |
| $T_1$ | $T_2$ | $S_1$ | $S_2$ |
| $T_2$ | $S_1$ | $S_2$ | $T_1$ |

The potency ratio was calculated using following formula:

**Concentration of unknown = $n_1/t_1 \times$ anti log $\{(S_1+S_2)-(T_1+T_2)/(S_2+T_2)-(S_1+T_1) \times \log n_2/n_1\}$ Cs**

n1 = Lower Standard dose
n2 = Higher Standard dose
$t_1$ = Lower Test dose
$t_2$= Higher test dose
S1 = Mean of response of std ($S_1$)
S2 = Mean of response of std ($S_2$)
$T_1$ = Mean of response of test ($t_1$)
$T_2$ = Mean response of test ($t_2$)

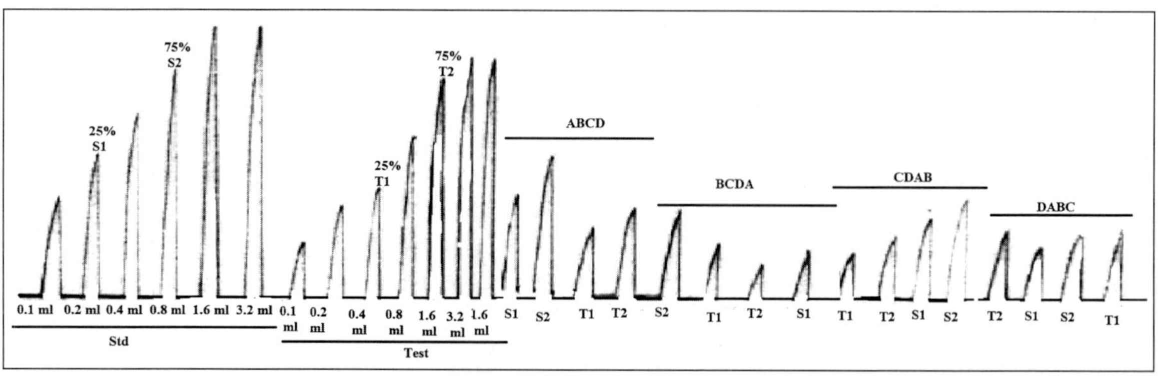


**Bioassay of oxytocin by using four point method.**

## Observation table:

| S.No. | Conc. of std. (μg/ml) | Type of Dose | Dose (ml) | Response height (mm) |
|---|---|---|---|---|
| 1. | | Standard | 0.1 | |
| 2. | | Standard | 0.2 ($S_1$) | |
| 3. | | Standard | 0.4 | |
| 4. | | Standard | 0.8 ($S_2$) | |
| 5. | | Standard | 1.6 | |
| 6. | | Standard | 3.2 | |
| 7. | | Test | 0.1 | |
| 8. | | Test | 0.2 | |
| 9. | | Test | 0.4 ($T_1$) | |
| 10. | | Test | 0.8 | |
| 11. | | Test | 1.6 ($T_2$) | |
| 12. | | Test | 3.2 | |
| 13. | | Test | 6.4 | |
| 14. | | $S_1$ | 0.2 | |
| 15. | | $S_2$ | 0.8 | |
| 16. | | $T_1$ | 0.4 | |
| 17. | | $T_2$ | 1.6 | |
| 18. | | $S_2$ | 0.8 | |
| 19. | | $T_1$ | 0.4 | |
| 20. | | $T_2$ | 1.6 | |
| 21. | | $S_1$ | 0.2 | |
| 22. | | $T_1$ | 0.4 | |
| 23. | | $T_2$ | 1.6 | |
| 24. | | $S_1$ | 0.2 | |
| 25. | | $S_2$ | 0.8 | |
| 26. | | $T_2$ | 1.6 | |
| 27. | | $S_1$ | 0.2 | |
| 28. | | $S_2$ | 0.8 | |
| 29. | | $T_1$ | 0.4 | |

## Precautions:

1. Cut out all the blood capillaries present on muscle preparation by using a sharp scissor.
2. Use thin piece (2-3cm) as it is more sensitive than bulky piece.
3. The level of PSS in the organ bath should remain constant throughout the experiment by marking the level with elastic ring/marker.
4. Speed of the drum should be slow (0.25mm) and the lever should be placed tangential to the drum.
5. The no. of washing and the interval between them should be kept constant.
6. Carefully mounting of the uterus preparation.
7. Organ bath containing de jalon solution maintained at 30-32°C

# VIVA-VOCE

**Q.1 What is mean by four point bioassay.**

**Ans:** This method is almost similar to the three point bioassay, but in this method 2 doses of the standard and the 2 doses of the test are used. The section of the standard doses should be such that they lie on the linear portion of the CRC and also the ratio between the smaller to greater dose should be preferably 1:2. The selection of the test doses is done by hit and trial method so that the responses fall on the linear part of the curve.

**Q.2 Which pattern is given in responses.**

**Ans:** The pattern of doses is

$$\begin{matrix} S_1 & S_2 & T_1 & T_2 \\ S_2 & T_1 & T_2 & S_1 \\ T_1 & T_2 & S_1 & S_2 \\ T_2 & S_1 & S_2 & T_1 \end{matrix}$$

**Q.3 Give the formula of four point bioassay.**

**Ans:**

Concentration of unknown = $n_1/t_1 \times$ anti log $\{(S_1+S_2)-(T_1+T_2)/(S_2+T_2)-(S_1+T_1) \times \log n_2/n_1\}$ Cs

# Experiment No. 14

## Object: To calculate pA2 value for atracurium using acetylcholine as agonist employing frog rectus abdominus muscle preparation.

## Principle:

The $pA_2$ value is devised by Sir Heinz Otto Schild in Quantitative Pharmacology. In1947 pA scale, to express drug antagonism.

pAx value is calculated to compare the potency of antagonists acting on the same receptor.

The pAx value is defined as the negative logarithm of the molar concentration of the antagonist required to reduce the effect of a multiple dose(x) of the agonist to that of a single dose in the absence of antagonist. The meaning of $pA_2$ is the affinity of the antagonist to the receptor. For antagonist, efficacy is 0 and affinity is one.

Higher the pAx value, more potent is the antagonist. The determination of $pA_2$ (X=2) and pA10 (X=10) values have wider applications. If the difference between these two values is found to be 0.95 or very near, the antagonism is likely to be of competitive type. An antagonist acting on the same receptor will have same $pA_2$ value in all the tissue or organ preparations.

## Requirements:

**Animal:** Frog

**Drugs:** Acetylcholine, atracurium

**Physiological solution:** Frog ringer

**Apparatus:** Student's single unit organ bath, aeration or oxygen delivery tube, isotonic frontal writing lever, fulcrum, Sherrington's recording drum, reservoir, pinch cork, screw clip etc.

## Experimental conditions:

Temperature: 30-32°C

Tension of lever: 0.5gm

Magnification: 10 times

Aeration: 70-72 bubble/min

## Procedure:

1. Pith or stun the frog and lay it on its back on the frog-dissecting board. Pin the four limbs.
2. Remove the skin on the abdomen and expose the rectus abdominus muscle.
3. Cut the muscle into small segments.
4. Tie a thread to the top and bottom of each muscle preparation before detaching the muscle from the body of the frog.
5. Mount the preparation in up-right position in the organ bath containing frog Ringer solution under a tension of 0.5 g. There is no need of maintaining the bath temperature since it is an amphibian tissue preparation. Bubble the organ with air.
6. Relax the tissue for 45 min, during which period wash the tissue with fresh quantum of ringer for at least four times.
7. Record the concentrations due to acetylcholine using either simple sideway or frontal writing lever. 90 second contact time and a total 5 min time cycle may be used for proper recording of the responses.
8. Record at least four responses to increasing doses of acetylcholine or till you get the maximum response. The maximum response is achieved if one gets same or slightly less response with a higher concentration.
9. Two doses bearing 1:2 dose ratios were selected and eliciting sub maximal responses (A, 2A) for $pA_2$ determination.
10. The tissue was standardized with the selected doses of acetylcholine.
11. A tissue is said to be standardized when it responds identically to the same dose of an agonist when repeated.
12. The concentration due to the double dose of acetylcholine (2A) were recorded in the presence of varying concentration ($B_1$, $B_2$, $B_2$) of atracurium.
13. The response due to double the dose of Ach (2A) i.e., before adding atracurium, as 100% response was considered.
14. The corresponding percent (%) response to this dose of Ach (2A) in the presence of varying concentration of atracurium was determined.
15. Graph was plotted representing negative log of molar concentration of atracurium employed along X-axis and % response along Y-axis.
16. $pA_2$ value is defined as the negative log of molar concentration of atracurium required reducing the effect of dose 2A to A, respectively.
17. The $pA_2$ value for atracurium was read directly from the graph. It corresponded to the percentage response obtained with half the dose of Ach (A).

Calculate $pA_2$ value of as follows:

$$pA_2 = -\log [B] + \log \{([A]_2/[A]_1)-1\}$$

Where $[B]$ = Molar concentration of antagonist.

$[A]_2 = EC_{50}$ of agonist in the presence of antagonist.

$[A]_1 = EC_{50}$ of agonist in the absence of antagonist.

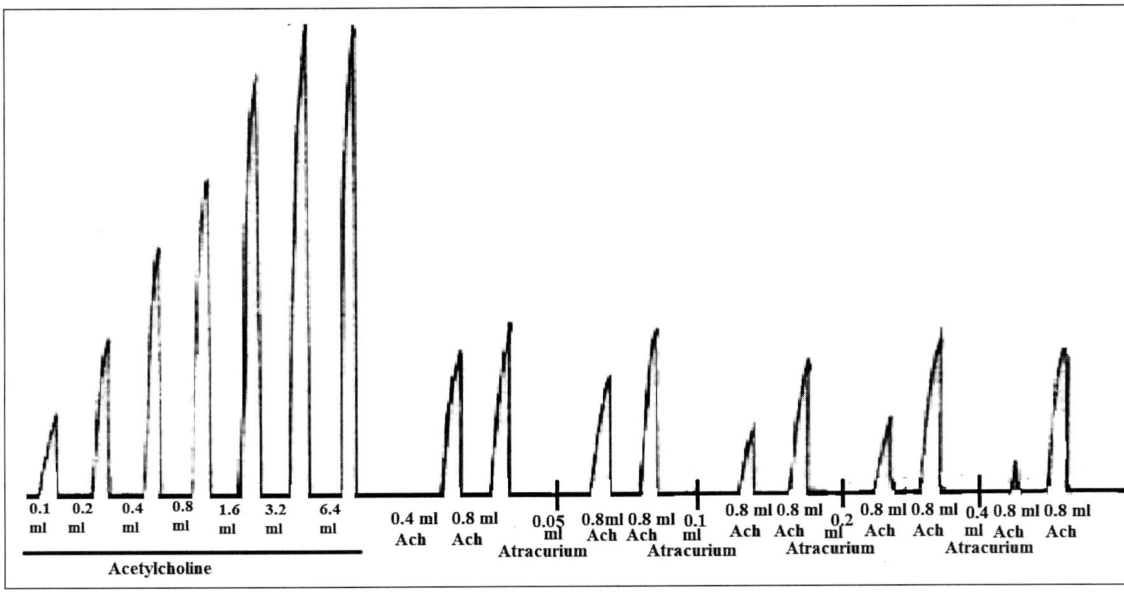


**pA2 value for atracurium using acetylcholine**

## Observation Table:

| S.No. | Type of dose | Dose (ml) | Concentration (µg) | Molar concentration | Response height (mm) | % Response height |
|---|---|---|---|---|---|---|
| 1. | | | | | | |
| 2. | | | | | | |
| 3. | | | | | | |
| 4. | | | | | | |
| 5. | | | | | | |
| 6. | | | | | | |

## Precautions:

1. Cut out all the blood capillaries present on muscle preparation by using a sharp scissor.
2. Use thin piece (2-3cm) as it is more sensitive than bulky piece.

3. The level of PSS in the organ bath should remain constant throughout the experiment by marking the level with elastic ring/marker.
4. Speed of the drum should be slow (0.25mm) and the lever should be placed tangential to the drum.
5. The no. of washing and the interval between them should be kept constant.
6. Organ bath containing frog ringer solution maintained at 30-32°C

## VIVA-VOCE

**Q.1 Define $pA_2$ value.**

**Ans:** The $pA_2$ value is defined as the negative logarithm of the molar concentration of the antagonist required to reduce the effect of a multiple dose(x) of the agonist to that of a single dose in the absence of antagonist.

**Q.2 Give formula of $pA_2$ value.**

**Ans:** Calculate $pA_2$ value of as follows:

$$pA_2 = -\log [B] + \log \{([A]_2/[A]_1)-1\}$$

Where $[B]$ = Molar concentration of antagonist.

$[A]_2 = EC_{50}$ of agonist in the presence of antagonist.

$[A]_1 = EC_{50}$ of agonist in the absence of antagonist.

# Experiment No. 15

## Object: To calculate pA2 value for atropine using acetylcholine as agonist using isolated guinea pig ileum preparation.

## Principle:

The pA**2** value is devised by Sir Heinz Otto Schild in Quantitative Pharmacology. In1947 pA scale, to express drug antagonism.

pAx value is calculated to compare the potency of antagonists acting on the same receptor.

The pAx value is defined as the negative logarithm of the molar concentration of the antagonist required to reduce the effect of a multiple dose(x) of the agonist to that of a single dose in the absence of antagonist. The meaning of pA2 is the affinity of the antagonist to the receptor. For antagonist, efficacy is 0 and affinity is one.

Higher the pAx value, more potent is the antagonist. The determination of pA2 (X=2) and pA10 (X=10) values have wider applications. If the difference between these two values is found to be 0.95 or very near, the antagonism is likely to be of competitive type. An antagonist acting on the same receptor will have same pA2 value in all the tissue or organ preparations.

## Requirements:

**Animal:** Guinea pig (400-600 gm)

**Drugs:** Acetylcholine, atropine

**Physiological solution:** Tyrode

**Apparatus:** Student's single unit organ bath, aeration or oxygen delivery tube, isotonic frontal writing lever, fulcrum, Sherrington's recording drum, reservoir, pinch cork, screw clip etc.

## Experimental conditions:

Temperature: 32-35°C

Tension of lever: 0.5gm

Magnification: 10 times

Aeration: 70-72 bubble/min

## Procedure:

1. The guinea pig is sacrificed by a blow on the head and carotid bleeding.
2. Cut open the abdomen and lift the caecum to ileo-caecal junction. Cut and remove a few centimeter long of the ileum portion and immediately place it in the watch glass containing tyrode solution.
3. Trim the mesentery and with gentle care clean the contents of the ileum by pushing the tyroide solution into the lumen of the ileum. Almost care should be taken to avoid any damage to the gut muscle.
4. Cut the ileum into small segments 2-3 cm long.
5. Take one piece of ileum of 2-3 cm long and tie a thread to the top and bottom ends without closing the lumen.
6. Mount the preparation in up-right position in the organ bath containing tyrode solution under a tension of 0.5 g. Tyrode solution maintained at 32-35°C. Bubble the organ with air.
7. Relax the tissue for 45 min, during which period wash the tissue with fresh quantum of ringer for at least four times.
8. Record the concentrations due to acetylcholine using either simple sideway or frontal writing lever. 90 second contact time and a total 5 min time cycle may be used for proper recording of the responses.
9. Record at least four responses to increasing doses of acetylcholine or till you get the maximum response. The maximum response is achieved if one gets same or slightly less response with a higher concentration.
10. Two doses bearing 1:2 dose ratios were selected and eliciting sub maximal responses (A, 2A) for $pA_2$ determination.
11. The tissue was standardized with the selected doses of acetylcholine.
12. A tissue is said to be standardized when it responds identically to the same dose of an agonist when repeated.
13. The concentration due to the double dose of acetylcholine (2A) were recorded in the presence of varying concentration ($B_1$, $B_2$, $B_2$) of atropine.
14. The response due to double the dose of Ach (2A) i.e., before adding atropine, as 100% response was considered.
15. The corresponding percent (%) response to this dose of Ach (2A) in the presence of varying concentration of atropine was determined.
16. Graph was plotted representing negative log of molar concentration of atropine employed along X-axis and % response along Y-axis.
17. $pA_2$ value is defined as the negative log of molar concentration of atropine required reducing the effect of dose 2A to A, respectively.

18. The $pA_2$ value for atropine was read directly from the graph. It corresponded to the percentage response obtained with half the dose of Ach (A).

Calculate $pA_2$ value of as follows:

$$pA_2 = -\log [B] + \log \{([A]_2/[A]_1)-1\}$$

Where $[B]$ = Molar concentration of antagonist.

$[A]_2 = EC_{50}$ of agonist in the presence of antagonist.

$[A]_1 = EC_{50}$ of agonist in the absence of antagonist.

## Observation Table:

| S.No. | Type of dose | Dose (ml) | Concentration (µg) | Molar concentration | Response height (mm) | % Response height |
|---|---|---|---|---|---|---|
| 1. | | | | | | |
| 2. | | | | | | |
| 3. | | | | | | |
| 4. | | | | | | |
| 5. | | | | | | |
| 6. | | | | | | |

## Precautions:

1. Cut out all the blood capillaries present on muscle preparation by using a sharp scissor.
2. Use thin piece (2-3cm) as it is more sensitive than bulky piece.
3. The level of PSS in the organ bath should remain constant throughout the experiment by marking the level with elastic ring/marker.
4. Speed of the drum should be slow (0.25mm) and the lever should be placed tangential to the drum.
5. The no. of washing and the interval between them should be kept constant.
6. Organ bath containing tyrode solution maintained at 32-35°C

# VIVA-VOCE

**Q.1 Define $pA_2$ value.**

**Ans:** The $pA_2$ value is defined as the negative logarithm of the molar concentration of the antagonist required to reduce the effect of a multiple dose(x) of the agonist to that of a single dose in the absence of antagonist.

**Q.2 Give formula of $pA_2$ value.**

**Ans:** Calculate $pA_2$ value of as follows:

$$pA_2 = -\log [B] + \log \{([A]_2/[A]_1)-1\}$$

Where [B] = Molar concentration of antagonist.

$[A]_2 = EC_{50}$ of agonist in the presence of antagonist.

$[A]_1 = EC_{50}$ of agonist in the absence of antagonist.

# Experiment No. 16

## Object: To determine $pD_2$ value of acetylcholine in the presence and absence of d-tubocurarine.

## Principle:

d-Tubocurarine is a neuromuscular blocking agent which blocks the nicotinic receptors in the skeletal muscle. As a result the actions of acetylcholine are inhibited in the presence of d-tubocurarine. The concentration response curve of acetylcholine will be shifted to the right in the presence of d-tubocurarine. Since the nature of the antagonism is of competitive type, the shift in the curve is parallel and there is no suppression in the maximal response of acetycholine.

The $EC_{50}$ values describe relative potency of the drugs, lower the value, more potent is the drug. Sometimes the same is expressed as $pD_2$ value which is defined as the negative log of molar concentration of the drug producing 50% of maximal response. Higher the $pD_2$ value, higher is the potency. In calculating the $pD_2$ value, the % of maximal response produced by each dose (concentration) is plotted against log molar concentration of the drug and the concentration producing 50% response is read as the $pD_2$ value. The $ED_{50}$ or $pD_2$ values are used to express the affinity of a drug. Both values can be interconvertible employing a simple equation i.e., if $ED_{50}$ expressed as ($m \times 10^{-n}$), $pD_2$=n-log m. Dose ratio ($EC_{50}$) is calculated by comparing the doses of acetylcholine that is required to produce 50% response in the presence and absence of d-tubocurarine. Note that the concentration of acetylcholine required to produced 50% response in the presence of d-tubocurarine is less as compared to per se effect of acetylcholine.

## Requirements:

**Animals:** Frog

**Drugs:** Acetylcholine (1 mg/ml), d-tubocurarine (1 mg/ml)

**Physiological solution:** Frog ringer

**Conditions:** Temperature: 37°C

Tension: 0.5gm

Magnification: 10 times

Aeration: 70-72 Bubble/min

## Procedure:

1. Pith or stun the frog and lay it on its back on the frog-dissecting board. Pin the four limbs.
2. Remove the skin on the abdomen and expose the rectus abdominus muscle.
3. Cut the muscle into small segments.
4. Tie a thread to the top and bottom of each muscle preparation before detaching the muscle from the body of the frog.
5. Mount the preparation in up-right position in the organ bath containing frog Ringer solution under a tension of 0.5 g. There is no need of maintaining the bath temperature since it is an amphibian tissue preparation. Bubble the organ with air.
6. Relax the tissue for 45 min, during which period wash the tissue with fresh quantum of ringer for at least four times.
7. Record the concentrations due to acetylcholine using either simple sideway or frontal writing lever. 90 second contact time and a total 5 min time cycle may be used for proper recording of the responses.
8. Record at least four responses to increasing doses of acetylcholine or till you get the maximum response. The maximum response is achieved if one gets same or slightly less response with a higher concentration.
9. Add d-tubocurarine (1mg/ml) to the reservoir containing frog ringer and irrigate the tissue with d-tubocurarine containing ringer for 30 min.
10. Repeat the concentration response curves of acetylcholine in the presence of d-tubocurarine.
11. Label and fix both the concentration response curves of acetylcholine, i.e. one in the absence and the other in the presence of d-tubocurarine. Calculate the relative $EC_{50}$ values and note the nature of antagonism.

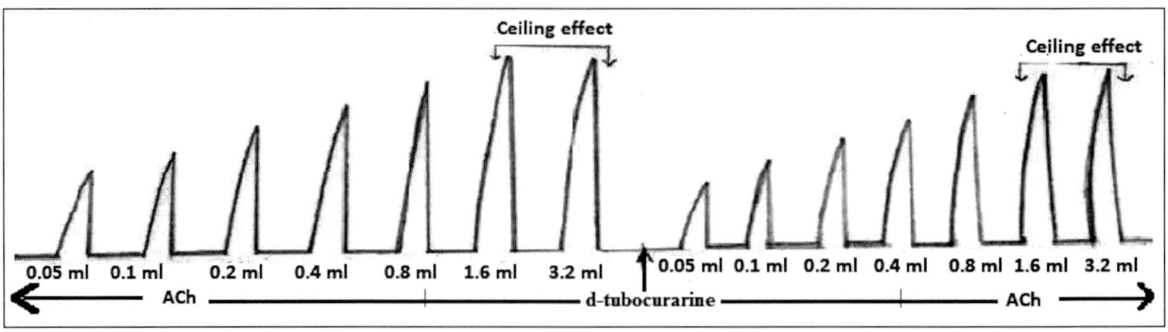


**$pD_2$ value of acetylcholine in the presence and absence of d-tubocurarine.**

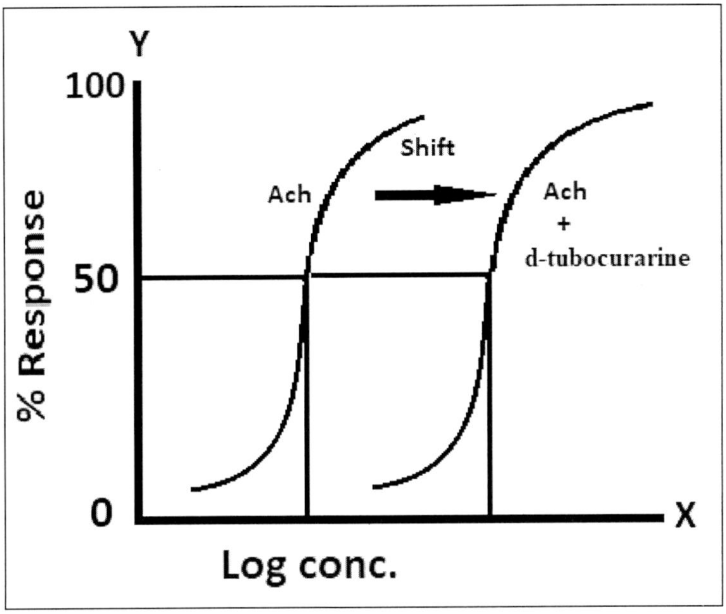


**pD2 value of acetylcholine in the presence and absence of d-tubocurarine.**

## Observation Table:

| S.No. | Dose of acetylcholine (ml) | Concentration (μg) | Log concentration | Response height (mm) without d-tubocurarine | % Response height | Molar concen-tration |
|---|---|---|---|---|---|---|
| 1. | 0.1 | 100 | 2 | | | |
| 2. | 0.2 | 200 | 2.301 | | | |
| 3. | 0.4 | 400 | 2.602 | | | |
| 4. | 0.8 | 800 | 2.903 | | | |
| 5. | 1.6 | 1600 | 3.204 | | | |
| 6. | 3.2 | 3200 | 3.505 | | | |
| | | | | | | |

| S.No. | Dose of acetylcholine (ml) | Concentration (µg) | Log concentration | Response height (mm) with d-tubocurarine | % Response height | Molar concen-tration |
|---|---|---|---|---|---|---|
| 1. | 0.1 | 100 | 2 | | | |
| 2. | 0.2 | 200 | 2.301 | | | |
| 3. | 0.4 | 400 | 2.602 | | | |
| 4. | 0.8 | 800 | 2.903 | | | |
| 5. | 1.6 | 1600 | 3.204 | | | |
| 6. | 3.2 | 3200 | 3.505 | | | |

$$\text{Dose ratio} = \frac{EC_{50} \text{ in the presence of d-tubocurarine}}{EC_{50} \text{ in the absence of d-tubocurarine}}$$

**Calculation:**

**% Height = Height in under consideration/Max. height x100**

$$\text{Molar concentration} = \frac{\text{Available concentration}}{\text{mol. wt. of Ach X 1000}}$$

$$\text{Available concentration} = \frac{\text{Dose in ml X Dose in µg}}{\text{Organ bath capacity}}$$

**From the graph find out the $EC_{50}$**

**From the $EC_{50}$ value find out the $pD_2$ value:**

$pD_2 = -\log (EC_{50})$

$= -\log (M \times 10^{-n})$

$= n - \log m$

## Precautions:

1. The level of ringer solution in the organ bath should remain constant throughout the experiment by marking the level with elastic ring/marker.
2. Speed of the drum should be slow (0.25mm) and the lever should be placed tangential to the drum.
3. The no. of washing and the interval between them should be kept constant.

# VIVA-VOCE

**Q.1 Define $pD_2$ value.**

**Ans:** $pD_2$ value which is defined as the negative log of molar concentration of the drug producing 50% of maximal response. Higher the $pD_2$ value, higher is the potency.

**Q.2 Give formula of $pD_2$ value.**

**Ans:** $pD_2 = -\log (EC_{50})$

**Q.3 Give the formula of molar concentration.**

**Ans:**

$$\text{Molar concentration} = \frac{\text{Available concentration}}{\text{mol. wt. of Ach X 1000}}$$

**Q.4 Give the formula of available concentration.**

**Ans:**

$$\text{Available concentration} = \frac{\text{Dose in ml X Dose in µg}}{\text{Organ bath capacity}}$$

# Experiment No. 17

## Object: To determine $pD_2$ value of histamine in the presence and absence of mepyramine.

## Principle:

Histamine is an autacoid having profound physiological effect in the body. Besides the triple response caused by it, histamine has spasmogenic response on intestinal smooth muscle. By acting on $H_1$ – histamine receptor it causes the contraction of intestinal smooth muscle. Guinea pig is highly sensitive to histamine. The guinea pig ileum preparation is very commonly used for isolated tissue work. It is sensitive to histamine in nanogram/ml concentrations. Mepyramine is a selective $H_1$ – histamine receptor antagonist. Overnight fasted animals are used to get better response of drugs on intestinal smooth muscle.

The $EC_{50}$ values describe relative potency of the drugs, lower the value, more potent is the drug. Sometimes the same is expressed as $pD_2$ value which is defined as the negative log of motar concentration of the drug producing 50% of maximal response. Higher the $pD_2$ value, higher is the potency. In calculating the $pD_2$ value, the % of maximal response produced by each dose (concentration) is plotted against log molar concentration of the drug and the concentration producing 50% response is read as the $pD_2$ value. The $ED_{50}$ or $pD_2$ values are used to express the affinity of a drug. Both values can be interconvertible employing a simple equation i.e., if $ED_{50}$ expressed as ($m \times 10^{-n}$), $pD_2$=n-log m. Dose ratio ($EC_{50}$) is calculated by comparing the doses of histamine that is required to produce 50% response in the presence and absence of mepyramine. Note that the concentration of histamine required to produced 50% response in the presence of mepyramine is less as compared to per se effect of histamine.

## Requirements:

**Animals:** Guinea pig

**Drugs:** Histamine (1 mg/ml), mepyramine (1 mg/ml)

**Physiological solution:** Tyrode

**Conditions:** Temperature: 37°C

Tension: 0.5gm

Magnification: 10 times

Aeration: 70-72 Bubble/min

## Procedure:

1. The guinea pig is sacrificed by a blow on the head and carotid bleeding.
2. Cut open the abdomen and lift the caecum to ileo-caecal junction. Cut and remove a few centimeter long of the ileum portion and immediately place it in the watch glass containing tyrode solution.
3. Trim the mesentery and with gentle care clean the contents of the ileum by pushing the tyrode solution into the lumen of the ileum. Almost care should be taken to avoid any damage to the gut muscle.
4. Cut the ileum into small segments 2-3 cm long.
5. Take one piece of ileum of 2-3 cm long and tie a thread to the top and bottom ends without closing the lumen.
6. Mount the preparation in up-right position in the organ bath containing tyrode solution under a tension of 0.5 g. Tyrode solution maintained at 32-35°C. Bubble the organ with air.
7. Relax the tissue for 45 min, during which period wash the tissue with fresh quantum of ringer for at least four times.
8. Record the concentrations due to histamine using either simple sideway or frontal writing lever. 90 second contact time and a total 5 min time cycle may be used for proper recording of the responses.
9. Record at least four responses to increasing doses of histamine or till you get the maximum response. The maximum response is achieved if one gets same or slightly less response with a higher concentration.
10. Add mepyramine (1mg/ml) to the reservoir containing tyrode and irrigate the tissue with mepyramine containing tyrode for 30 min.
11. Repeat the concentration response curves of histamine in the presence of mepyramine.
12. Label and fix both the concentration response curves of histamine, i.e. one in the absence and the other in the presence of mepyramine. Calculate the relative $EC_{50}$ values and note the nature of antagonism.

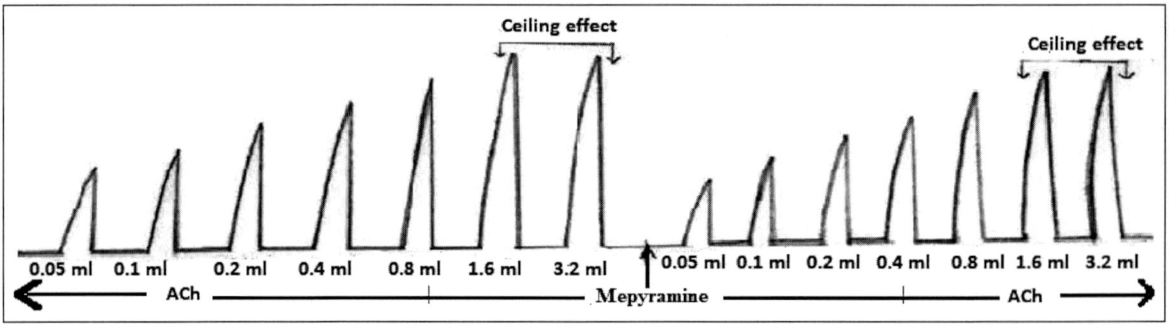


**pD2 value of histamine in the presence and absence of mepyramine.**

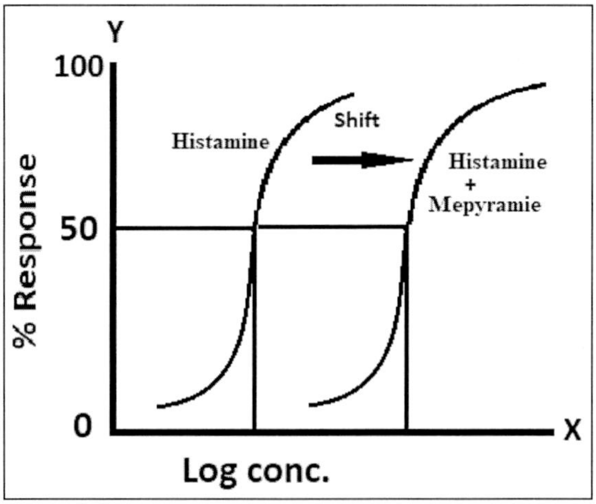


**pD2 value of histamine in the presence and absence of mepyramine.**

## Observation Table:

| S.No. | Dose of acetylcholine (ml) | Concentration (µg) | Log concentration | Response height (mm) without mepyramine | % Response height | Molar concen-tration |
|---|---|---|---|---|---|---|
| 1. | 0.1 | 100 | 2 | | | |
| 2. | 0.2 | 200 | 2.301 | | | |
| 3. | 0.4 | 400 | 2.602 | | | |
| 4. | 0.8 | 800 | 2.903 | | | |
| 5. | 1.6 | 1600 | 3.204 | | | |
| 6. | 3.2 | 3200 | 3.505 | | | |
| | | | | | | |

| S.No. | Dose of acetylcholine (ml) | Concentration (μg) | Log concentration | Response height (mm) with mepyramine | % Response height | Molar concen-tration |
|---|---|---|---|---|---|---|
| 1. | 0.1 | 100 | 2 | | | |
| 2. | 0.2 | 200 | 2.301 | | | |
| 3. | 0.4 | 400 | 2.602 | | | |
| 4. | 0.8 | 800 | 2.903 | | | |
| 5. | 1.6 | 1600 | 3.204 | | | |
| 6. | 3.2 | 3200 | 3.505 | | | |

$$\text{Dose ratio} = \frac{EC_{50}\text{ in the presence of mepyramine}}{EC_{50}\text{ in the absence of mepyramine}}$$

**Calculation:**

**% Height = Height in under consideration/Maximum Height x100**

$$\text{Molar concentration} = \frac{\text{Available concentration}}{\text{mol. wt. of Ach X 1000}}$$

$$\text{Available concentration} = \frac{\text{Dose in ml X Dose in μg}}{\text{Organ bath capacity}}$$

**From the graph find out the $EC_{50}$**

**From the $EC_{50}$ value find out the $pD_2$ value:**

$pD_2 = -\log (EC_{50})$

$= -\log (M \times 10^{-n})$

$= n - \log m$

## Precautions:

1. The level of ringer solution in the organ bath should remain constant throughout the experiment by marking the level with elastic ring/marker.
2. Speed of the drum should be slow (0.25mm) and the lever should be placed tangential to the drum.
3. The no. of washing and the interval between them should be kept constant.

# VIVA-VOCE

**Q.1 Define $pD_2$ value.**

**Ans:** $pD_2$ value which is defined as the negative log of molar concentration of the drug producing 50% of maximal response. Higher the $pD_2$ value, higher is the potency.

**Q.2 Give formula of $pD_2$ value.**

**Ans:** $pD_2 = -\log (EC_{50})$

**Q.3 Give the formula of molar concentration.**

**Ans:**

$$\text{Molar concentration} = \frac{\text{Available concentration}}{\text{mol. wt. of Ach X 1000}}$$

**Q.3 Give the formula of concentration.**

**Ans:**

$$\text{Available concentration} = \frac{\text{Dose in ml X Dose in µg}}{\text{Organ bath capacity}}$$

# Experiment No. 18

## Object: To determine $pD_2$ value of acetylcholine in the presence and absence of atropine using isolated rat colon prepration.

## Principle:

Rat ileum is an intestinal smooth muscle. Acetylcholine causes the contraction of the smooth muscle by acting on muscarinic receptors. Atropine blocks muscarinic receptors in the smooth muscle. Therefore, atropine blocks acetylcholine induced contraction in rat ileum. The concentration response curve of acetylcholine will be shifted to the right in the presence of atropine. The nature of antagonism is of competitive type and thus surmountable.

The spontaneous contractions of the preparation can be reduced by reducing the calcium content in physiological salt solution and maintaining the bath at room temperature. The muscle (colon) preparation obtained from an unstarved rat gives more stable contraction.

The $EC_{50}$ values describe relative potency of the drugs, lower the value, more potent is the drug. Sometimes the same is expressed as $pD_2$ value which is defined as the negative log of motar concentration of the drug producing 50% of maximal response. Higher the $pD_2$ value, higher is the potency. In calculating the $pD_2$ value, the % of maximal response produced by each dose (concentration) is plotted against log molar concentration of the drug and the concentration producing 50% response is read as the $pD_2$ value. The $ED_{50}$ or $pD_2$ values are used to express the affinity of a drug. Both values can be interconvertible employing a simple equation i.e., if $ED_{50}$ expressed as ($m \times 10^{-n}$), $pD_2$=n-log m. Dose ratio ($EC_{50}$) is calculated by comparing the doses of acetylcholine that is required to produce 50% response in the presence and absence of d-tubocurarine. Note that the concentration of acetylcholine required to produced 50% response in the presence of d-tubocurarine is less as compared to per se effect of acetylcholine.

## Requirements:

**Animals:** Rat

**Drugs:** Acetylcholine (1 mg/ml), atropine (1 mg/ml)

**Physiological solution:** Modified ringer

**Conditions:** Temperature: 37°C

Tension: 0.5gm

Magnification: 10 times

Aeration: 70-72 Bubble/min

## Procedure:

1. Sacrifice the animal by cervical dislocation.
2. Cut open the abdomen and identify the colon. The right flexure, i.e., the subhepatic region of the colon where the ascending colon turns to become the transverse colon, is cut out and placed in a shallow dish containing modified ringer solution.
3. The lumen is gently cleaned and a 3 cm long tissue is mounted in the organ bath containing modified ringer solution under a tension of 0.5 g. Bubble the organ with air.
4. Relax the tissue for 45 min, during which period wash the tissue with fresh quantum of ringer for at least four times.
5. Record the concentrations due to acetylcholine using either simple sideway or frontal writing lever. 90 second contact time and a total 5 min time cycle may be used for proper recording of the responses.
6. Record at least four responses to increasing doses of acetylcholine or till you get the maximum response. The maximum response is achieved if one gets same or slightly less response with a higher concentration.
7. Add atropine (1mg/ml) to the reservoir containing frog ringer and irrigate the tissue with atropine containing ringer for 30 min.
8. Repeat the concentration response curves of acetylcholine in the presence of atropin.
9. Label and fix both the concentration response curves of acetylcholine, i.e. one in the absence and the other in the presence of atropine. Calculate the relative $EC_{50}$ values and note the nature of antagonism.

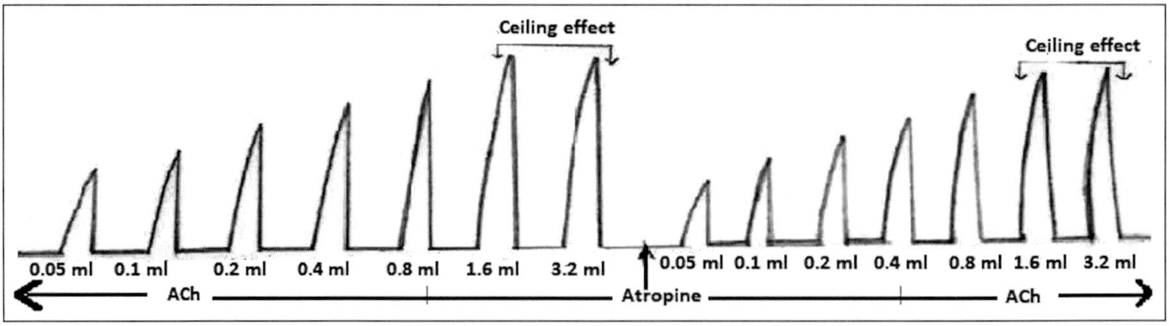


**pD2 value of acetylcholine in the presence and absence of atropine**

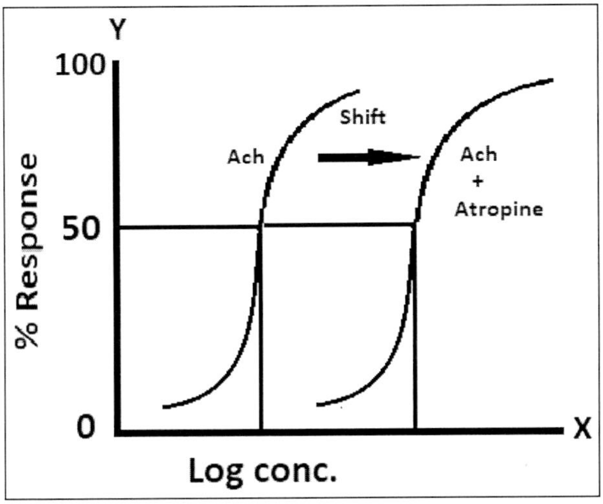


**pD2 value of acetylcholine in the presence and absence of atropine**

## Observation Table:

| S.No. | Dose of acetylcholine (ml) | Concentration (µg) | Log concentration | Response height (mm) without atropine | % Response height | Molar concentration |
|---|---|---|---|---|---|---|
| 1. | 0.1 | 100 | 2 | | | |
| 2. | 0.2 | 200 | 2.301 | | | |
| 3. | 0.4 | 400 | 2.602 | | | |
| 4. | 0.8 | 800 | 2.903 | | | |
| 5. | 1.6 | 1600 | 3.204 | | | |
| 6. | 3.2 | 3200 | 3.505 | | | |

| S.No. | Dose of acetylcholine (ml) | Concentration (µg) | Log concentration | Response height (mm) with atropine | % Response height | Molar concentration |
|---|---|---|---|---|---|---|
| 1. | 0.1 | 100 | 2 | | | |
| 2. | 0.2 | 200 | 2.301 | | | |
| 3. | 0.4 | 400 | 2.602 | | | |
| 4. | 0.8 | 800 | 2.903 | | | |
| 5. | 1.6 | 1600 | 3.204 | | | |
| 6. | 3.2 | 3200 | 3.505 | | | |

$$\textbf{Dose ratio} = \frac{EC_{50} \text{ in the presence of atropine}}{EC_{50} \text{ in the absence of atropine}}$$

**Calculation:**

**% Height = Height in under consideration/Max. height x100**

$$\textbf{Molar concentration} = \frac{\text{Available concentration}}{\text{mol. wt. of Ach X 1000}}$$

$$\textbf{Available concentration} = \frac{\text{Dose in ml X Dose in µg}}{\text{Organ bath capacity}}$$

**From the graph find out the $EC_{50}$**

**From the $EC_{50}$ value find out the $pD_2$ value:**

$pD_2 = -\log (EC_{50})$

$= -\log (M \times 10^{-n})$

$= n - \log m$

## Precautions:

1. The level of ringer solution in the organ bath should remain constant throughout the experiment by marking the level with elastic ring/marker.
2. Speed of the drum should be slow (0.25mm) and the lever should be placed tangential to the drum.
3. The no. of washing and the interval between them should be kept constant.

## VIVA-VOCE

**Q.1 Define $pD_2$ value.**

**Ans:** $pD_2$ value which is defined as the negative log of molar concentration of the drug producing 50% of maximal response. Higher the $pD_2$ value, higher is the potency.

**Q.2 Give formula of $pD_2$ value.**

**Ans: $pD_2 = -\log (EC_{50})$**

**Q.3 Give the formula of molar concentration.**

**Ans:**

$$\text{Molar concentration} = \frac{\text{Available concentration}}{\text{mol. wt. of Ach X 1000}}$$

**Q.3 Give the formula of concentration.**

**Ans:**

$$\text{Available concentration} = \frac{\text{Dose in ml X Dose in } \mu\text{g}}{\text{Organ bath capacity}}$$

# Experiment No. 19

## Object: To study the effects of various spasmogenic and spasmolytic drugs on intestine of rabbit.

## Principle:

Spasmogenic- The drugs, which produce spasm, are called as spasmogens. Spasmogens are also called as spasmodic, spasmogenics.

Ex:- Acetylcholine, Barium chloride

Relaxants- The drugs, which relieves the spasm of the smooth muscles by producing relaxation of smooth muscles. Relaxants are also called as antispasmodics, spasm relaxants and spasmolytics.

Ex:- Atropine, Adrenaline

## Requirements:

**Animal**: Rabbit

**Equipment**: Reservoir, tubing, haemostatic forceps, isolated organ bath, aeration tube, isotonic frontal writing lever and recording drum.

**Drugs:** Acetylcholine (10 µg/ml), $BaCl_2$ (20 µg/ml)

**Conditions:** Temperature: 37°C

Tension: 0.5gm

Magnification: 10 times

Aeration: 70-72 Bubble/min

PSS: Tyrode solutions

## Procedure:

1. Give a midline incision on the abdomen and expose the whole abdomen.
2. Dissect out and transfer the piece of small intestine in a petridish containing tyrode solution at a room temperature, which is constantly supplied with aeration.
3. Place one end of intestine over the tip of the pipette and apply the air pressure, to wash out the contents. (Use the intestine directly, if animal has not been fed recently.)

4. Pass a thread to both the ends of intestine by inserting a needle from the inner side of the intestine.
5. Tie one end of the intestine to aeration tube and other end to the frontal writing lever.
6. Balance the weight of 0.5 gm on the lever by using piece of plasticin wax. (Balance the lever by putting the weight at the end of the shorter arms and mark the point of tissue attachment.)
7. Follow the time cycle given below for the recording the response of intestine of rabbit.
   5 minutes time cycle:
   i. 30 seconds- Take the base line record.
   ii. 90 seconds- Allow the drug to contact with tissue.
   iii. 120 seconds- Give the first wash
   (Give three subsequent washings at the interval of 1 min.)
   iv. 300 seconds- Give the second dose.
8. Inject the doses into the organ tube containing tyrode solution and intestine preparation as given in the observation table.
9. After completion of doses, label and fix the graph with fixing solution.

## Observation table:

| S.No. | Drug | Dose | Tone and force of contraction | Response (Height of contraction in mm) |
|---|---|---|---|---|
| 1. | Tyrode solution | | | |
| 2. | Acetylcholine | | | |
| 3. | Barium chloride | | | |
| 4. | Atropine<br>+<br>Acetylcholine | | | |
| 5. | Adrenaline | | | |

## Precautions:

1. Avoid the use of forceps to transfer the intestine, because it damages the tissue, handle it by fingers.
2. Avoid the application of excessive air pressure.
3. Use about 2-3 cm piece of intestine for the experimental purpose.

# VIVA-VOCE

**Q.1 Define Spasmogenic.**

**Ans:** The drugs, which produce spasm, are called as spasmogens. Spasmogens are also called as spasmodic, spasmogenics.

**Q.2 Define spasmolytics.**

**Ans:** The drugs, which relieves the spasm of the smooth muscles by producing relaxation of smooth muscles. Relaxants are also called as antispasmodics, spasm relaxants and spasmolytics.

**Q.3 How acetylcholine produces spasmogenic action.**

**Ans:** It produces tone of force of contraction of smooth muscle of intestine.

# Experiment No. 20

## Object: To study the carrageenan-induced anti-inflammatory activity on acute paw edema in rats.

## Principle:

Inflammation is a tissue –reaction to infection, injury, irritation or foreign substance. It is a part of the host defence mechanism but when it becomes uncontrolled it is a hopeless condition. Aging is also considered to be an inflammatory response. There are several tissue factors or mechanisms that are known to be involved in the inflammatory reactions such as release of histamine, bradykinin and prostaglandins.

The development of non-steroidal anti-inflammatory agents in recent years has contributed a lot in not only overcoming the human suffering such as arthritis but also has helped in understanding the tissue mechanism of inflammation

Carrageenan-induced paw edema is the most commonly used method in experimental pharmacology. Carrageenan is a sulphate polysaccharide obtained from sea weed (Rhodophyceae), and by causing the release of histamine, 5-HT,bradykinin and prostaglandins, it produces inflammation and edema.

This method is based upon the ability of anti-inflammatory agents to inhibit the edema produced in the hind paw of the rat after injection of a phlogistic agent (carragennan). The volume of the injected paw is measured before and after the application of irritants. The paw volume of treated animals is compared with control. Plethysmograph is used to measure paw volume. Plethysmograph, (simple apparatus containing mercury. The mercury displacement due to dipping of the paw can be directly read from scale attached to the mercury column or adjusting the mercury level in the arm B to the original level by moving the arm B up/down and note the volume required in both the arms equal)

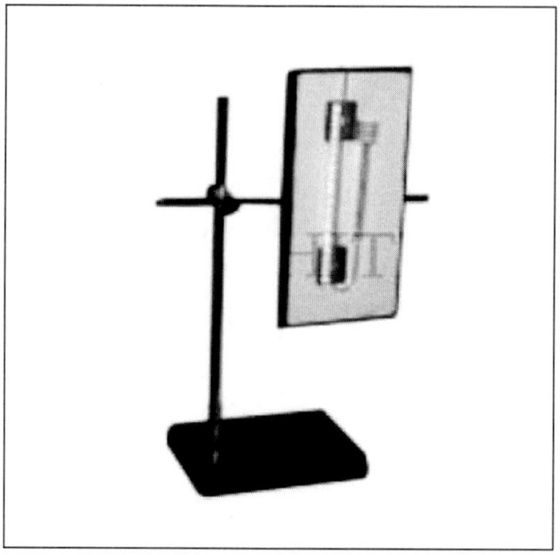

**Plethysmometer**

## Requirements:

**Animal**: Rats, (150-200g)

**Equipment**: Plethysmograph, syringe and needle

**Drugs:** Carrageenan (1% w/v solution and inject 0.1 ml underneath the plantar region). Indomethacin (Dose 20 mg/kg, s.c, Prepare a stock solution containing 4mg/ml of the drug and inject 0.5 ml/100 g of body weight of the animal).

## Procedure:

1. Weigh the animals and number them.
2. Mark a mark on both the hind paws (right and Left) just beyond tibio-tarsal junction, so that every time the paw is dipped in the mercury column upto the fixed mark to ensure constant paw volume.
3. Note the initial paw volume (both right and left) of each rat by mercury displacement method.
4. Divide the animals into two groups each comprising of at least six rats. To one group inject saline and to the second group inject indomethacin subcutaneously.
5. After 30 min inject 0.1 ml of 1% (w/v) carragenan in the plantar region of the left paw of control as well as indomethacin –treated group. The right paw will serve as reference non-inflammed paw for comparison.

6. Note the paw volume of both legs of control and indomethacin-treated rats at 15,30,60,and 120 min after carragenan challenge.
7. Calculate the percent difference in the right and left paw volumes of each animal of control and indomethacin –treated group. Compare the mean percent change in paw colume in control and drug –treated animals and express as per cent edema inhibition by the drug.

## Observation table:

| S.No. | Body wt. (gm) | Treatment | Dose (mg/kg) | Paw volume (ml) as measured by mercury displacement at | | | | | | | | | |
|---|---|---|---|---|---|---|---|---|---|---|---|---|---|
| | | | | 0 | | 15 | | 30 | | 60 | | 120 | |
| | | | | R | L | R | L | R | L | R | L | R | L |
| 1. | | Control | | | | | | | | | | | |
| 2. | | Control | | | | | | | | | | | |
| 3. | | Control | | | | | | | | | | | |
| 4. | | Control | | | | | | | | | | | |
| 5. | | Control | | | | | | | | | | | |
| 6. | | Control | | | | | | | | | | | |
| **Mean** | | | | | | | | | | | | | |
| **% difference in R and L** | | | | | | | | | | | | | |
| 1. | | Indomethacine | | | | | | | | | | | |
| 2. | | Indomethacine | | | | | | | | | | | |
| 3. | | Indomethacine | | | | | | | | | | | |
| 4. | | Indomethacine | | | | | | | | | | | |
| 5. | | Indomethacine | | | | | | | | | | | |
| 6. | | Indomethacine | | | | | | | | | | | |
| **Mean** | | | | | | | | | | | | | |
| **% difference in R and L** | | | | | | | | | | | | | |

R = Right paw; L = Left paw. Inject 0.1 ml of 1% (w/v) carrageenan 30 min after indomethacin.

## Precautions:

1. Note the initial paw volume (both right and left) of each rat by mercury displacement method.
2. Properly inject 0.1 ml underneath the plantar region.

## VIVA-VOCE

**Q.1 How does cause carrageenan inflammation.**

**Ans:** Carrageenan is a sulphate polysaccharide obtained from sea weed (Rhodophyceae), and by causing the release of histamine, 5-HT,bradykinin and prostaglandins, it produces inflammation and edema.

**Q.2 Explain Plethysmograph.**

**Ans:** A plethysmograph is an instrument for measuring changes in volume within an organ or whole body (usually resulting from fluctuations in the amount of blood or air it contains).

**Q.3 Define inflammation.**

**Ans:** Inflammation is a tissue –reaction to infection, injury, irritation or foreign substance. It is a part of the host defence mechanism but when it becomes uncontrolled it is a hopeless condition. Aging is also considered to be an inflammatory response.

# Experiment No. 21

## Object: To study the croton oil induced anti-inflammatory activity on ear edema in mice.

## Principle:

Croton oil-induced ear oedema is an acute animal model of inflammation. The method has developed primarily as a bioassay for the concentration assessment of the antiphlogistic and thymolytic activities of topically applied steroids. Croton oil (crotonisoleum), is obtained from the seeds of croton tiglium, a tree belonging to the natural order Euphorbiaceae, and native or cultivated in India and the Malay islands. When applied to the skin, croton oil acts as a powerful irritant, inducing inflammation. The mechanism of croton oil induced inflammation involves an increase in phospholipase $A_2$ activity that in turn leads to the release of arachidonic acid and subsequently biosynthesis of leukotriene's and prostaglandins, the important mediators in inflammatory processes.

## Requirements:

**Animal**: Male mice (20-25 gm)

**Equipment**: Surgical scissors, blade, micropipette (10µg), analytical balance.

**Drugs:** Dexamethasone (1.6 µg/10 ul of the solvent system). Solvent system [Pyridine: warter: acetone (P:W:A) in the ratio of 4:2:14] Croton oil (1% v/v) in P:W:A solution, ethyl ether as an anesthetic agent. Prepare the solution fresh and keep in ice.

## Procedure:

1. Weight and number the animals. Randomize the animals into different groups according to the body weights.
2. Anaesthetize the animals using ethyl ether as an anesthetic agent.
3. Hold the animal gently from front paws and apply 10ul of dexamethasone solution to the left inner ear of the mouse and allow it to dry at room temperature. Similarly, apply 10 ug of solvent system to the right ear of the mice that serves as control for comparison with the left ear. For control group, apply the solvent to both the left and right inner ears.
4. After two hours of the treatment, apply 10ul of croton oil solution (1% v/v) to the left inner ear of each animal. The right ear (solvent applied) (P:W:A) would serve as control.

5. After six hours of the croton oil application, sacrifice all the animals under $Co_2$ anesthesia and excise both the ears with the help of sharp scissor or blade. Weight both left and right ears of each animal separately on an analytical balance.
6. Note the difference in the weights of treated (steroid) and untreated (control) ears.
7. Calculate the % increase in ear weights of each animals in a group. Take the mean of the whole group.

$$\% \text{ increase in ear weight} = \frac{\text{Wt. of left ear} - \text{Wt. of right ear}}{\text{Wt. of right ear}} \times 100$$

8. Calculate the % decrease in ear edema due to steroid application as compared to solvent control group.

$$\% \text{ inhibition of ear edema} = \frac{\text{Mean \% increase in ear weight solvent treated group} - \text{Mean \% increase in ear Wt. of steroid treated group}}{\text{Mean \% increase in ear weight of solvent treated group}} \times 100$$

## Observation table:

| S.No. | Treatment | Dose | Animal ID | Body wt. (gm) | Wt. of right ear (mg) (solvent) | Wt. of left ear (mg) (croton oil) | % increase in ear wt. | % inhibiton |
|---|---|---|---|---|---|---|---|---|
| 1. | Solvent control | | 1 | | | | | |
| | | | 2 | | | | | |
| | | | 3 | | | | | |
| | | | 4 | | | | | |
| | | | 5 | | | | | |
| | | | 6 | | | | | |
| | | | Mean | | | | | |
| | | | SEM | | | | | |
| 2. | Dexamethasone | 1.6 µg/ 10 ul of PWA | 1 | | | | | |
| | | | 2 | | | | | |
| | | | 3 | | | | | |
| | | | 4 | | | | | |
| | | | 5 | | | | | |
| | | | 6 | | | | | |
| | | | Mean | | | | | |
| | | | SEM | | | | | |

## Precautions:

1. Hold animal properly.
2. Properly apply 10 ul of croton oil solution.
3. Sacrifice animal under $Co_2$ anesthesia.

# VIVA-VOCE

**Q.1 Role of croton oil in ear edema model.**

**Ans:** Croton oil-induced ear oedema is an acute animal model of inflammation. The method has developed primarily as a bioassay for the concentration assessment of the antiphlogistic and thymolytic activities of topically applied steroids.

**Q.2 Write down the MOA of croton oil induced inflammation.**

**Ans:** The mechanism of croton oil induced inflammation involves an increase in phospholipase $A_2$ activity that in turn leads to the release of arachidonic acid and subsequently biosynthesis of leukotriene's and prostaglandins, the important mediators in inflammatory processes.

**Q.3 What is the role of dexamethasone.**

**Ans:** Dexamethasone is a steroid that prevents the release of substances in the body that cause inflammation. Dexamethasone is used to treat many different conditions such as allergic disorders, skin conditions, ulcerative colitis, arthritis, lupus, psoriasis, or breathing disorders.

**Q.4 Give formula of percentage of inhibition of ear edema.**

**Ans:**

$$\text{\% inhibition of ear edema} = \frac{\text{Mean \% increase in ear weight solvent treated group} - \text{Mean \% increase in ear Wt. of steroid treated group}}{\text{Mean \% increase in ear weight of solvent treated group}} \times 100$$

# Experiment No. 22

## Object: To study the analgesic effect of Diclofenac sodium in albino rats by using analgesiometer (Tail-flick method).

## Principle:

Pain is an unpleasant feeling, which make us uncomfortable and reduce the physical as well as mental alertness. Although pain are also useful for us because it acts as a warning signal and it warns about something uncommon inside or outside our body. If the pain is minor it may be tolerated but if the pain becomes severe it has to be managed at earliest.

Analgesia is defined as a state of reduced awareness to pain and analgesics are substances which decrease pain sensation (pain –killers) by increasing threshold to painful stimuli.

The commonly used analgesics are aspirin, paracetamol (non-narcotic type) and morphine (narcotic type).

Painful reaction in experimental animals can be applying noxious (unpleasant) stimuli such as:

(i) Thermal (radiant heat as a source of pain)
(ii) Chemical (irritants such as acetic acid and bradykinin)
(iii) Physical pressure (tail compression)

In the laboratory commonly used procedures are tail-flick (tail-withdrawal from the radiant heat source) method using analgesiometer, eddy's hot plate (jumping from the hot plate at 55 ° C) method and acetic acid –induced writhing.

## Requirements:

**Animals:** Albino rat (150-200 gm)

**Drugs:** Diclofenac sodium (11mg/kg, i.m.), Normal saline (0.9%w/v NaCl solution)

**Equipment:** Analgesiomete

**Other:** Animal cage, balance to weight small animals, syringes, stop watch etc.

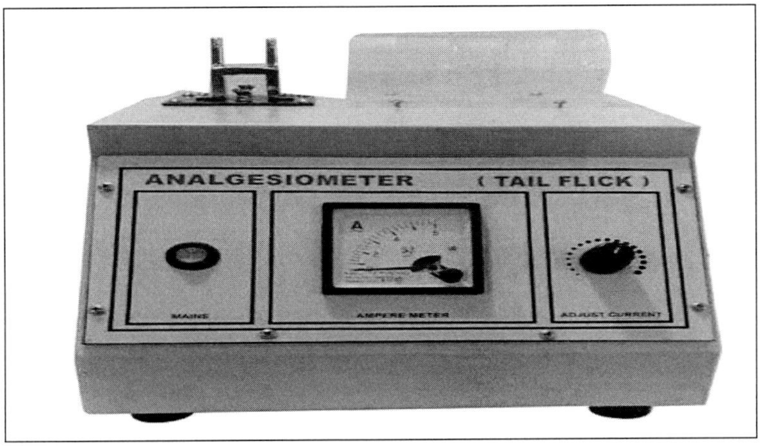


**Analgesiometer (Tail-flick method)**

## Procedure:

1. Weigh the animals, divided them into two groups and mark them.
2. Take basal reaction time to radiant heat by placing the tip (last 1-2 cm) of the tail on the radiant heat source.
3. The tail-withdrawal from the heat (flicking response) is taken as the end point.
4. Normally a rat withdraws its tail within 3-5 sec. A cut off period of 10-12 sec is observed to prevent damage to the tail. Any animal failing to withdraw its tail in 3-5 sec is rejected from the study. Take at least 3-5 basal reaction times for each rat at a gap of 5min to confirm normal behaviour of the animal.
5. Inject normal saline to the control group and diclofenac sodium to the standard group in the specified dose and note the reaction time after 5, 15, 30 and 60 min after the drug. As the reaction time reaches 10 sec it is considered maximum analgesia and the tail is removed from the source of heat to avoid tissue damage.
6. Calculate percentage increase in reaction time (index of analgesia) at each time interval.

## Observation table:

| Animal | Treatment | Basal reaction time (sec) | | | | | Reaction time (sec) after treatment | | | |
|---|---|---|---|---|---|---|---|---|---|---|
| | | 1 | 2 | 3 | 4 | 5 | 5min | 15min | 30min | 60min |
| 1. | Control | | | | | | | | | |
| 2. | Control | | | | | | | | | |
| 3. | Control | | | | | | | | | |

| Animal | Treatment | Basal reaction time (sec) | | | | | Reaction time (sec) after treatment | | | |
|---|---|---|---|---|---|---|---|---|---|---|
| | | 1 | 2 | 3 | 4 | 5 | 5min | 15min | 30min | 60min |
| 4. | Control | | | | | | | | | |
| 5. | Control | | | | | | | | | |
| 6. | Control | | | | | | | | | |
| 7. | Standard | | | | | | | | | |
| 8. | Standard | | | | | | | | | |
| 9. | Standard | | | | | | | | | |
| 10. | Standard | | | | | | | | | |
| 11. | Standard | | | | | | | | | |
| 12. | Standard | | | | | | | | | |

**Group I: Control (Normal saline: 0.9% w/v NaCl solution)**

**Group II: Standard (Diclofenac sodium: 11mg/kg, i.m.)**

## Precautions:

1. Handle the animal carefully and restrain it.
2. Accurately drug concentration as per animal body weight.
3. A cut-off period of 10-12 sec is observed to prevent the damage to the tail.

## VIVA-VOCE

**Q.1 Write down the principle of tail flick analgesiometer.**

**Ans:** Radiant heat by placing the tip (last 1-2 cm) of the tail on the radiant heat source. The tail-withdrawal from the heat (flicking response) is taken as the end point. Normally a rat withdraws its tail within 3-5 sec. A cut off period of 10-12 sec is observed to prevent damage to the tail. Any animal failing to withdraw its tail in 3-5 sec is rejected from the study. Take at least 3-5 basal reaction times for each rat at a gap of 5min to confirm normal behaviour of the animal.

**Q.2 Define pain.**

**Ans:** Pain is an unpleasant feeling, which make us uncomfortable and reduce the physical as well as mental alertness.

**Q.3 Define analgesia.**

**Ans:** Analgesia is defined as a state of reduced awareness to pain and analgesics are substances which decrease pain sensation (pain –killers) by increasing threshold to painful stimuli.

**Q,4 Give method in analgesic activity of drug using central and peripheral methods.**

**Ans:** Centrally- Tail-flick (tail-withdrawal from the radiant heat source), eddy's hot plate (jumping from the hot plate at 55 ° C)

Peripheral- acetic acid –induced writhing test, Carrageenan-induced paw edema test.

# Experiment No. 23

## Object: To study the analgesic effect of Morphine on mice by using analgesiometer (Hot plate method).

### Principle:

In this method head is used as a source of pain. Animals are individually placed on a hot plate maintained at constant temperature (55°C) and the reaction of animals, such as paw licking or jump response is taken as the end point. Analgesics increase the reaction time. The method was first describe by Eddy and Leimbach (1953).

Pain is an unpleasant feeling, which make us uncomfortable and reduce the physical as well as mental alertness. Although pain are also useful for us because it acts as a warning signal and it warns about something uncommon inside or outside our body. If the pain is minor it may be tolerated but if the pain becomes severe it has to be managed at earliest.

Analgesia is defined as a state of reduced awareness to pain and analgesics are substances which decrease pain sensation (pain –killers) by increasing threshold to painful stimuli.

The commonly used analgesics are aspirin, paracetamol (non-narcotic type) and morphine (narcotic type).

Painful reaction in experimental animals can be applying noxious (unpleasant) stimuli such as:

(i) Thermal (radiant heat as a source of pain)
(ii) Chemical (irritants such as acetic acid and bradykinin)
(iii) Physical pressure (tail compression)

### Requirements:

**Animal**: Mice (20-25 g)

**Equipment**: Eddy's hot plate

**Drugs:** Morphine sulphate (dose 5 mg/kg, s.c, prepare a stock solution containing 0.5 mg/ml and inject 1 ml/100 g of body weight of mouse)

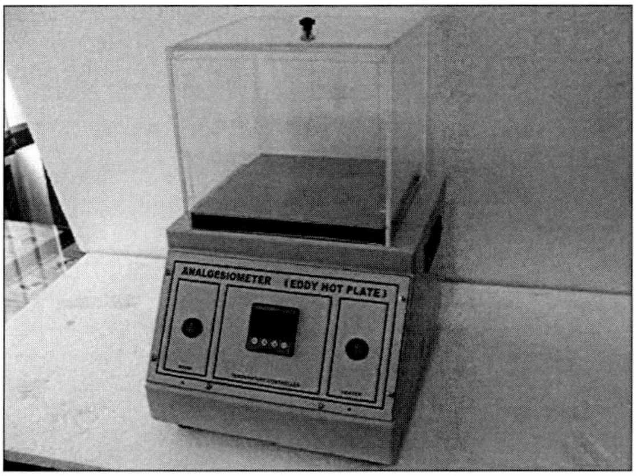


**Eddy's Hot Plate**

## Procedure:

1. Weigh and number the mice.
2. Take the basal reaction – time by observing hind paw licking or jump response (whichever appears first) in animals when placed on the hot plate maintained at constant temperature (55° C). Normally animals show such response in 6-8 sec. A cut off period of 15 sec is observed to avoid damage to the paws.
3. Inject morphine to animals and note the reaction time of animals on the hot plate at 15, 30, 60 and 120 min after the drug administration. As the reaction time increases with morphine, 15 sec is taken as maximum analgesia and the animals are removed from the hot plate to avoid injury to the paws.
4. Calculate percent increase in reaction time (as index of analgesia) at each time interval.

## Observation time:

| S.No. | Basal reaction time (sec) | | Reaction time (sec) after morphine administration | |
|---|---|---|---|---|
| | Paw-licking | Jump response | Paw-licking | Jump response |
| 1. | | | | |
| 2. | | | | |
| 3. | | | | |
| 4. | | | | |
| 5. | | | | |
| 6. | | | | |

## Precautions:

1. Handle the animal carefully and restrain it.
2. Accurately drug concentration as per animal body weight.
3. A cut-off period of 13-15 sec is observed to prevent the damage to the paws.

## VIVA-VOCE

**Q.1 Write down the principle of Hot plate analgesiometer.**

**Ans:** In this method head is used as a source of pain. Animals are individually placed on a hot plate maintained at constant temperature (55°C) and the reaction of animals, such as paw licking or jump response is taken as the end point.

**Q.2 Define pain.**

**Ans:** Pain is an unpleasant feeling, which make us uncomfortable and reduce the physical as well as mental alertness.

**Q.3 Define analgesia.**

**Ans:** Analgesia is defined as a state of reduced awareness to pain and analgesics are substances which decrease pain sensation (pain –killers) by increasing threshold to painful stimuli.

**Q,4 Give method in analgesic activity of drug using central and peripheral methods.**

**Ans:** Centrally- Tail-flick (tail-withdrawal from the radiant heat source), eddy's hot plate (jumping from the hot plate at 55 ° C)

Peripheral- acetic acid –induced writhing test, Carrageenan-induced paw edema test.

# Experiment No. 24

## Object: To study the analgesic effect of drug on mice by using acetic acid induced writhing test in mice.

## Principle:

Writhing is abdominal constriction response cause by intraperitoneal injection of phenylquinone, bradykinin, acetic acid or any irritant like turpentine etc. In this response the belly of animal touches ground, hind legs are stretched backwards and there are abdominal constrictions. Intraperitoneal injection of acetic acid or any irritant like turpentine produces pain reaction which gives writhing response. The writhing effect consists of abdominal constriction, turning of trunk (twist) and extension of hind legs (stretching) response by the animal is taken as reaction to chemically induced pain. Centrally and peripherally acting analgesics are the drug which is narcotic and non-narcotic type inhibits writhing response in animals.

## Requirements:

**Animals:** Mice (25-30 g)

**Drugs**: Morphine sulphate (dose 5 mg/kg, s.c. prepare a stock solution containing 0.5 mg/ml and inject 1 ml/100 g of body weight of mouse), acetic acid (1%v/v Inject 1 ml/100 g of body weight of the animal).

## Procedure:

1. Weigh and number the mice.
2. Divide the animals into two groups, each consisting of 5 animals.
3. Administer appropriate volume of acetic acid solution to the first group (which serves as control), place them individually under glass jar for observation.
4. Note the onset on wriths. Record the number of abdominal contractions, trunk twist response and extension of hind limbs as well as the number of animals showing such response during a period of 10 min.
5. To the second group of animals inject morphine. Fifteen minutes later, administer acetic acid solution to these animals. Note the onset and severity of writhing response as done in step 4.

6. Calculate the mean writhing scores in control and morphine treated groups. Note the inhibition of pain response by morphine.
7. Analgesic activity can be expressed by percent maximal possible effect (%MPE).

$$\%MPE = \frac{\text{Mean wriths in treated group} - \text{Mean control wriths}}{\text{Cut off time (shown)} - \text{Mean control wriths}} \times 100$$

## Observation table:

| S.No. | Body Wt. (gm) | Treatment | No. of wriths (10 min) | Responders (n/n) |
|---|---|---|---|---|
| 1. | | Control (Acetic acid) | | |
| 2. | | Control (Acetic acid) | | |
| 3. | | Control (Acetic acid) | | |
| 4. | | Control (Acetic acid) | | |
| 5. | | Control (Acetic acid) | | |
| | | Mean | | |
| 1. | | Morphine + Acetic acid | | |
| 2. | | Morphine + Acetic acid | | |
| 3. | | Morphine + Acetic acid | | |
| 4. | | Morphine + Acetic acid | | |
| 5. | | Morphine + Acetic acid | | |
| | | Mean | | |

## Precautions:

1. Doses are carefully calculated.
2. Handle the animal carefully and restrain it.
3. A cut-off period of 13-15 sec. is observed to prevent the damage to the tail.

## VIVA-VOCE

**Q.1 What is mean by writhing test.**

**Ans:** Writhing test is a chemical method used to induce pain of peripheral origin by injection of irritant principles like phenylquinone, acetic acid in mice. Analgesic activity of the test compound is inferred from decrease in the frequency of writhing's.

**Q.2 Explains writhing inducing agents.**

**Ans:** Writhing test is a chemical method used to induce pain of peripheral origin by injection of irritant principles like phenylquinone, acetic acid in mice. Writhing's generated by parenteral administration of acetic acid in mice, are due to profound pain of endogenous nature which recur for a prolonged period of time.

**Q3. How to observe writhing in rats.**

**Ans:** Writhing is defined as a stretch, tension to one side, extension of hind legs, or contraction of the abdomen so that the abdomen of the mice touches the floor, or turning of the trunk.

# Pharmacology-III
## (Semester-VI)

# Experiment No. 1

## Object: Dose calculation in pharmacological experiments.

## Theory:

Experimental animals are very important tool in non-human research models. Dosage calculations and stock solution preparation based on dosage rationable formula are prerequisites to drug administration in experimental animals.

However, drug dosage calculations and stock solutions preparations are not clearly explained in most scientific literature.

## Vehicle of choice, drugs dissolutions & volume selections rationale:

A vehicle is any substance that are used as medium for drug administration. Vehicle which is an essential consideration in all animal research should be biologically inert, it has non toxic effects on animals.

Eg-water, normal saline (0.9% NaCl), 50% polyethylene glycol, 5-10% tween 80, 0.25% methyl cellulose (or) carboxy methyl cellulose.

In most researches involving experimental animals dosage are usually calculated from stock solution of the test drugs dissolved in vehicle. According to OECD's (organization of economic corporation and development) guidelines, dosage of drug should be constituted in an appropriate volume not usually exceeding 10 ml/kg body weight of experimental animals for non aqueous solvent in oral route of administration. However in the case of aqueous solvents, 20ml/kg body weight can be considered (OECD, 2000). Large dose volume (40ml/kg body weight) can cause unnecessary stress to animals and can also overload the stomach capacity and pass immediately into the small bowel or can result in passive reflux in stomach, aspiration, pneumonia, pharyngeal, esophageal and gastric irritation or injury with structure formation, esophageal and gastric rupture and stress.

However, highly viscous drug solutions should be diluted whenever possible, for ease of administration.

However, final dilution volume should be not exceed 20ml/kg. based on 10ml/kg volume selection, required dose volume for a 100gm rat can be calculated as follows 100g/1000g x10ml= 1ml

**Table 1: OECD guidelines on volume selection**

| Standard volume | Body weight of animals | Calculated volume on the base of body weight of animals in ml |
|---|---|---|
| 10 ml/kg (appropriate value) | 100 | 1.00 |
| | 120 | 1.20 |
| | 130 | 1.30 |
| | 140 | 1.40 |
| | 150 | 1.50 |
| 20 ml/kg (maximum volume) | 100 | 2.00 |
| | 120 | 2.40 |
| | 130 | 2.60 |
| | 140 | 2.80 |
| | 150 | 3.00 |

## 1. Dose calculation and preparation of stock solution of a standard drug for experimental animals.

Diclofenac is a standard drug used in animal model of screening for agents with anti inflammatory activity at standard doses ranging between 10 mg/kg to 25 mg/kg body weight.

Example I. calculate the required dose of diclofenac for a rat weighing 150 g at a standard dose 10 mg/kg (Label claim- 50 mg/kg)

**1st step**: Dosage calculation

$$\text{Required dose for 150 gm rat} = \frac{\text{Body weight of rats (gm)}}{\text{1000 gm}} \times \text{Standard dose (mg)}$$

$$= \frac{\text{150 gm}}{\text{1000 gm}} \times \text{10 mg}$$

$$= \text{1.5 mg}$$

**2nd step**: Dissolution of diclofenac in a suitable volume of vehicle for oral administration

From the above calculation, 150 g rat requires 3.25 mg of diclofenac and this dosage (1.5 mg) should be constituted in not more than 1.5 ml of normal saline according to the OECD's guideline.

In general 150 gm rats requires 1.5 mg dose in 1.5 ml vehicle

Then, one tablet of sylimarin (70 mg) would be constituted in

Then 1 tablet of diclofenac would be dissolve in

$$= \frac{1.5 \text{ ml}}{1.5 \text{ mg}} \times 50 \text{ mg}$$

$$= 50 \text{ ml}$$

Finally $= 50 \text{ ml} / 50\text{mg}$

$$= 1 \text{ mg/ml}$$

In above stock solution contain 1 mg diclofenac per ml

According OECD guidelines rational for administration of drug for varying body weight are as follows:

**Table 2: Stock solution preparation for diclofenac tablet and required doses for animals of different body weights.**

| Standard dose | Stock solution | Animals body weight | Calculated dose(mg) | Equivalent dose in ml |
|---|---|---|---|---|
| 10 mg/kg | 50 mg in 50 ml (1mg/ml) | 120 | 1.2 | 1.2 |
| | | 125 | 1.25 | 1.25 |
| | | 130 | 1.3 | 1.3 |
| | | 140 | 1.4 | 1.4 |
| | | 150 | 1.5 | 1.5 |

## 2. Dose calculation and preparation of stock solution for salt or bulk compound

Streptozotocin (STZ) is a inducer for diabetes in experimental animals at a standard dose of 70 mg/kg for rat via intraperitoneal route.

The required dose of steptozotocin to induce experimental diabetes intraperitoneally in a rat weighing 180 gm at a standard dose of 70 mg/kg can be calculated as follows Formula

$$\text{Required dose for 180 gm rat} = \frac{\text{Body weight of rats (gm)}}{1000 \text{ gm}} \times \text{Standard dose (mg)}$$

$$= \frac{180 \text{ gm}}{1000 \text{ gm}} \times 70 \text{ mg}$$

$$= 12.6 \text{ mg}$$

It means for 180 gm of rats requires 12.6 mg of STZ

According OECED recommended volume for intraperitoneally administration is ranging between 2 ml/kg to 5 ml/kg

Based on 2 ml/ kg volume selection for STZ we requires

180 gm animal requires 0.36 ml volume

Therefore bulk stock of STZ could be prepared of more animal by weighing 200 mg (02 gm) of STZ

$$= \frac{0.36\text{ ml}}{12.6\text{ mg}} \times 200\text{ mg} = 5.71\text{ ml of vehicle volume}$$

It means 35.02 mg STZ per ml in above stock solution

**Table 3: Stock solution preparation for STZ and required doses for animals of different body weights.**

| Standard dose | Stock solution | Animals body weight | Calculated dose(mg) | Equivalent dose in ml |
|---|---|---|---|---|
| STZ<br>70 mg/kg | 200 mg in<br>5.71 ml<br>(35.02 mg/ml) | 150 | 10.5 | 0.30 |
| | | 160 | 11.2 | 0.32 |
| | | 180 | 12.6 | 0.36 |
| | | 200 | 14 | 0.40 |
| | | 220 | 15.4 | 0.44 |

## 3. Dosage calculation and preparation of stock solution of crude plant extract for experimental animals

With reference to table 1 above, stock solutions and doses of a plant extract 300 mg/kg for a rat weighing 150 g be calculated as follows;

**Step 1:** Dosage calculation

Body weight of animal = 150 gm

$$\text{Required dose for 150 gm rat} = \frac{\text{Body weight of rats (gm)}}{1000\text{ gm}} \times \text{Standard dose (mg)}$$

$$= \frac{150\text{ gm}}{1000\text{ gm}} \times 300\text{ mg}$$

$$= 45\text{ mg}$$

**Step 2:** Dissolution of dose in a suitable vehicle for oral administration

From the OECD's guidelines,

150 gm rat requires 45 mg of the crude plant extract which should be constituted in not more than 1.5 ml of normal saline (see table 1 above) according to the OECD guideline.

150 gm = 45 mg = 1.5 ml of normal saline.

Bulk volume of the stock solution required for large number of animals can be calculated by multiplying both sides by a constant value as follows;

45 mg = 1.5 ml

10 x 45 mg = 10 x 1.5 ml

450 mg = 15 ml

450 mg of crude plant extract will be dissolved in 15 ml of normal saline

It means stock solution contain 30 mg/ ml crude extract

**Table 4: Stock solutions from selected doses of a crude plant extract**

| Standard dose | Stock solution | Animals body weight | Calculated dose(mg) | Equivalent dose in ml |
|---|---|---|---|---|
| Plant extract 300 mg/kg | 450 mg in 15 ml (30 mg/ml) | 100 | 30 | 1.00 |
| | | 120 | 36 | 1.20 |
| | | 130 | 39 | 1.30 |
| | | 150 | 45 | 1.50 |
| | | 180 | 54 | 1.80 |

## 4. Dosage calculation and preparation of stock solution for Ampoules

Cisplatin is an anticancer drug used to induce hepatotoxicity in experimental animals (rats and mice) at a standard dose of 5 mg/kg (via intraperitoneal route)

The required dose of cisplatin to induce experimental hepatotoxicity intraperitoneally in rat weighing 100 gm at a standard dose of 5 mg/kg can be calculated as follows;

**Step 1: Dose calculation**

$$\text{Required dose for 100 gm rat} = \frac{\text{Body weight of rats (gm)}}{\text{1000 gm}} \times \text{Standard dose (mg)}$$

$$= \frac{\text{100 gm}}{\text{1000 gm}} \times \text{5 mg}$$

$$= \text{0.5 mg}$$

**Step 2: Required volume calculation for intraperitoneal injection**

From the above calculation, 100 g rat requires 0.5 mg of cisplatin and this dosage (0.5 mg) can be withdrawn directly from the stock of cisplatin which is present as 50 mg/50 ml (1 mg/ml) ampoule.

For 100 gm rats requires - = 1ml/1mg x 0.5 mg = 0.5 ml of Cisplatin

**Tablet 5: The required dose (volume) of cisplatin injection required for rats and mice of varying body weights.**

| Standard dose | Stock solution | Animals body weight | Calculated dose(mg) | Equivalent dose in ml |
|---|---|---|---|---|
| Cisplatin 70 mg/kg | 50 mg in 50 ml (1 mg/ml) | 100 | 0.5 | 0.5 |
| | | 120 | 0.6 | 0.6 |
| | | 150 | 0.75 | 0.75 |
| | | 180 | 0.6 | 0.9 |
| | | 200 | 1 | 1 |

## 5. Direct calculation of animals' dose from human dose

Some experimental situation may arise, when animal doses of compounds of different formulations (syrup, tonic, solution, ampoule injection, suspension and tablet) are calculated from average adult (70 kg) human dose.

For examples paracetamol syrup

Adult dose of paracetamol syrup is 10 ml 3 times a day for 70 kg adult = 10 x 3 = 30 ml per day

Dose for a rat weighing 200 g can be calculated as follows

70 kg (70,000 gm) adult man requires = 30 ml of paracetamol syrup per day,

Thus

$$\text{Required dose for 200 gm rat} = \frac{30\text{ ml}}{7000\text{ gm}} \times 200\text{ gm}$$

$$= 0.085\text{ ml}$$

Since the volume is very small to be measured with one ml syringe, it is recommended to dilute it for ten times (x10) Serial dilution for the paracetamol syrup.

Diluting 1 ml of paracetamol syrup with 9 ml of normal saline

Required new volume of paracetamol syrup for 200 gm rat from the diluted paracetamol syrup will be = 0.085 ml x10 = 0.85 ml

## Precautions

1. Before starting the experiment clean the apparatus and glassware.
2. Take accurate weight of drug on calibrated weighing balance.
3. Weigh the animal accurately on animal weighing balance.
4. Make all the stock solution in aseptic condition.
5. Make sure accurate volume should be injected in animal.

## VIVA-VOCE

**Q.1 Write down the full form of OECD.**

**Ans:** Organisation for Economic Co-operation and Development.

**Q.2 What is importance of dose calculation in experimental pharmacology.**

**Ans:** Dosage calculation in experimental pharmacology, involving the use of experimental animals is important in screening and development of new drugs. Dose calculation important for inject accurate dose in animal used in experiment.

**Q.3 Define stock solution.**

**Ans:** A stock solution is a concentrated solution that will be diluted to some lower concentration for actual use.

**Q.4 Which are the different parameters required for dose calculations.**

**Ans:** In experimental pharmacology following factors are important during dose calculation

i. Weight of animal
ii. Selection of vehicle
iii. Volume of injection in animal
iv. Label claim of drug
v. Final dose injection in animal

# Experiment No. 2

## Object: To study Anti-allergic activity by mast cell stabilization assay.

## Principle:

Mast cells or mastocytes are vital for the immune surveillance of the human body. These large connective tissue cells originate in the hematopoietic progenitor cells and are present in various tissues such as the skin, mucosa of the lungs, and digestive tract, as well as in the mouth, conjunctiva and nose. When activity by antigen, mast cells initiate subcellular signal transduction pathways and histamine, resulting in progression of allergic responses. Moreover, mast cells release certain prostaglandins and leukotrienes that contribute to the immediate inflammatory response. Mast cell stabilizers are thus important for prevention of different types of allergic and inflammatory reactions.

## Requirements:

**Animal:** Mice (30-40gm)

**Drugs and chemicals:** Disodium chromoglycate, 0.9% saline solution, RPMI 1640 buffer medium, 1% Toludine blue, egg albumin.

**Instruments:** Microscope with lens, centrifuge

## Procedure:

1. Mice are divided into two groups each containing three animals
2. A three days treatment schedule is followed.
   Group I received vehicle (5 ml/kg, i.p.).
   Group-II received standard drug Disodium chromoglycate (50 mg/kg, i.p.).
3. On fourth day of experiment animals are injected with 10 ml/kg of 0.9% saline solution into peritoneal cavity.
4. After this by gentle massage peritoneal fluid are collect after five minute and transfer into test tube containing 8-10 ml RPMI 1640 buffer medium (pH 7.2-7.4).
5. Then solution is then centrifuge at 400-500 rpm.
6. Discard the supernatant and wash the pellets of mast cells with same buffer medium twice by centrifugation.
7. The cell suspension challenge with egg albumin (100 mg/ml) and incubate at $37^0$ c for 10 minute

8. Finally cell suspension are stained with 1% toludine blue and observe under microscope.
9. Total 100 cells are counted from different visual areas.
10. Percent protection against degranulations are calculated.

## Observation table:

| Group | Total no. of cells (n=100) | |
|---|---|---|
| | **Granulated** | **Degranulated** |
| Vehicle treated | | |
| Disodium chromoglycate | | |

## Conclusion:

Pretreatment of animals with standard drugs stabilizes mast cell membrane and generates nitric oxide defensive mechanism that inhibits the release of chemokines which are responsible for vasoconstriction.

## Precautions:

1. Inject accurate dose of standard drug in animals.
2. Stain cell suspension carefully.
3. Care to be taken during centrifugation.
4. Observe cell under microscope carefully.

## VIVA-VOCE

**Q.1 What is mean by mast cell stabilizers.**

**Ans:** Mast cell stabilizers are medications used to prevent or control certain allergic disorders. They block mast cell degranulation, stabilizing the cell and thereby preventing the release of histamine and related mediators.

**Q.2 The role of mast cells in allergic inflammation.**

**Ans:** Mast cells interact directly with bacteria and appear to play a vital role in host defense against pathogens. Mast cells also have a central role in the initiation of the allergic immune response, that is providing signals inducing IgE synthesis by B-lymphocytes and inducing Th2 lymphocyte differentiation.

# Experiment No. 3

## Object: To study the anti-ulcer activity of a drug using pylorus ligand (SHAY) rat model.

## Theory:

Pylori ligation in rats leads to accumulation of gastric acid in the stomach leading to acute gastric ulceration. First demonstrated by Shay and co-workers in 1945. Peptic ulcer disease refers to pathological lesions and ulcers of any portion of gastrointestinal tract exposed to acid activated pepsin. Gastric ulcer refers to ulcer in the stomach where as duodenal ulcer is a ulcer found in duodenum of small intestine. Helicobacter pylori infection, a spiral shaped type of bacteria, is present in more than 90% of the patients with intestinal ulcers and more than 80% of patients with stomach ulcers.

## Requirements:

**Animals:** Albino wistar rats of weighing between 150-180 gm

**Drug and chemicals:** Anesthetic ether, Ranitidine, Normal saline

**Reagents:** Phenolphthalein, 0.1 N NaoH, Tofer's reagents

**Instruments:** Microscope, surgical instruments, pH meter

## Procedure:

1. Take rats weighing between 150-180gm in weight and divided into 2 groups each containing 4 rats.
2. Group 1 rats inject with normal saline and group 2 rats inject with ranitidine (20 mg/kg) orally.
3. Removed feed and water from animals before 24 hours.
4. 30 min prior to ligation ranitidine should be given.
5. Under light ether anesthesia midline abdominal incision is made and pylorus will be ligated with proper care and the wound is closed.
6. The rats are to be placed individually in separate cage and feed and water removes and allow them to recover.
7. After 4 hours sacrifice the animals, open the stomach with greater curvature, remove stomach contents and wash with isotonic saline solution.

8. Observe the formed ulcer under 10x magnification of microscope.
9. Finally calculate the ulcer index.

Ulcer score 1 mm= 1, 1-2 mm 2, > 2 mm33, >3 mm= 4

**Ulcer index=** (U1+ U2+ U3)* $10^{-1}$

U1- Average number of ulcer per animals

U2- Average of severity score

U3- % of animals with ulcer

Intensity of ulcer with scoring

0- Normal coloration, 0.5- red coloration, 1- spot ulcer, 1.5- hemorrhagic stress, 2- deep ulcer, 3- perforations.

## Observation tables:

| S.No. | Group | Ulcer index |
|---|---|---|
| 1. | Group 1 | |
| 2. | Group 2 | |

## Conclusion:

By comprising ulcer index of group shows anti-ulcer potency of test drug. Decrease in volume of gastric acid, free contents and total acidity means test drug has anti-secretary activity. Increase in pH shows drug has neutralizing activity.

## Precautions:

1. The abdomen was opened by a small midline incision below the xiphoid process.
2. Pylorus portion of stomach was slightly lifted out and ligated.
3. Precaution was taken to avoid traction to the pylorus or damage to its blood supply.
4. The stomach was placed carefully in the abdomen and the wound was sutured by interrupted sutures.

## VIVA-VOCE

**Q.1 Define ulcer.**

**Ans:** A disruption of the mucosal integrity of the stomach and/or duodenum leading to a local defect or excavation due to active inflammation.

**Q.2 Write down the principle of pylorus ligand (SHAY) rat model.**

**Ans:** Pylori ligation in rats leads to accumulation of gastric acid in the stomach leading to acute gastric ulceration. First demonstrated by Shay and co-workers in 1945. Peptic ulcer disease refers to pathological lesions and ulcers of any portion of gastrointestinal tract exposed to acid activated pepsin. Gastric ulcer refers to ulcer in the stomach where as duodenal ulcer is a ulcer found in duodenum of small intestine. Helicobacter pylori infection, a spiral shaped type of bacteria, is present in more than 90% of the patients with intestinal ulcers and more than 80% of patients with stomach ulcers.

**Q.3 What is advantages and disadvantage of pylorus ligation in rat.**

**Ans:** Advantages: Evaluates anti-ulcer drugs with various mechanisms of action and different doses.

Disadvantages: The ulcers localized in antrum of the stomach.

# Experiment No. 4

## Object: To study the anti-ulcer activity of a drug using NSAIDS induced ulcer model.

### Theory:

Peptic ulcer defined as an ulceration of the mucous membrane of the stomach, duodenum or esophagus. The imbalanced secretions of gastric acid, pepsin and duodenal mucosal defense mechanisms are the causes of such ulcers. Excessive non- steroidal and anti-inflammatory drugs (NSAIDs) consumption of can cause damage of gastrointestinal mucosa leading to ulcers. Aim of this experiment is to screen the drugs for their antiulcer activity.

### Requirements:

**Animals:** rats of weighing between 200-300 gm

**Drug and chemicals:** Ranitidine, Aspirin

### Procedure:

1. Take rats weighing between 200-300gm in weight and divided into 2 groups each containing 3 rats.
2. Group 1 rats inject with vehicle and group 2 rats inject with ranitidine (30 mg/kg) orally.
3. Both group administer with aspirin (30 mg/kg) after 30 minutes of administration of drug.
4. Remove feed and water from animals.
5. After 6 hours sacrifice the animals, open the stomach with greater curvature, remove stomach contents and wash with isotonic saline solution.
6. Observe the formed ulcer and measure the ulcer length.
7. Finally calculate the ulcer index.

Ulcer score 1 mm= 1, 1-2 mm3 2, > 2 mm3 3, >3 mm= 4

**Ulcer index=** (U1+ U2+ U3) * $10^{-1}$

U1- Average number of ulcer per animals

U2- Average of severity score

U3- % of animals with ulcer

Intensity of ulcer with scoring

1- Normal coloration, 0.5- red coloration, 1- spot ulcer, 1.5- hemorrhagic stress, 2- deep ulcer, 3- perforations.

## Observation tables:

| S.No. | Group | Ulcer index |
|---|---|---|
| 1. | Group 1 | |
| 2. | Group 2 | |

## Conclusion:

By comprising ulcer index of group shows anti-ulcer potency of test drug. Decrease in volume of gastric acid, free contents and total acidity means test drug has anti-secretary activity. Increase in pH shows drug has neutralizing activity.

## Precautions:

1. Inject accurate dose of NSAIDS in rat to induce ulcer.
2. Avoid feed and water to animals during experiment.
3. Carefully remove stomach content.
4. Accurately measure the ulcer length.

## VIVA-VOCE

### Q.1 Define ulcer.

**Ans:** A disruption of the mucosal integrity of the stomach and/or duodenum leading to a local defect or excavation due to active inflammation.

### Q.2 How do NSAIDs cause ulcer disease.

**Ans:** Excessive non- steroidal and anti-inflammatory drugs (NSAIDs) consumption of can cause damage of gastrointestinal mucosa leading to ulcers.

# Experiment No. 5

## Object: To study the effect of drugs on gastrointestinal motility.

### Theory:

The motility function gastrointestinal tract (GIT) is associated with

1. Forward propulsion of ingested food
2. Digestion
3. Absorption of nutrients and
4. Expulsion of unabsorbed food material.

These functions are adequately, supported by cyclic motor activity occurring in almost all parts of the GIT which is due to migrating my electrical complex (MMC) through electrical activity of the GIT. Any discrepancy in motility patter can affect, functionality of the GIT. A decrease in motility can lead to the stasis of food/chime in the intestine which favors the increases in the quantum of bacterial growth and cause constipation. Sometimes such situation may cause medical emergency when the barrier is breached, leading to bacterial translocation to other organs of the body. On the other hand, increased motility interferes with the digestion and absorption process and can lead to diarrhea and the malabsorption syndrome. The clinically known conditions of motility disorders such as achalasia, gastric stasis, outlet obstruction, acute intestinal ileum, chronic intestinal pseudo obstruction, magacolon, and, generalized disorders of motility deserve treatment with safer drugs. The evaluation of gastrointestinal (GI) motility is helpful in

1. Determining the therapeutic potential of new drugs in motility disorders,
2. Determining alteration in motility secondary to physiological or pharmacological 42 stimuli.
3. Evaluating the effect of pathological condition on GI transit.

In vivo methods in animals exhibit true effects of investigational drugs in biological milieu. Studies of motility of GI are associated with observation of marker in immediately excised sections of GIT or observation of motility in conscious animals using electrical gadgets. The following are the most popular in vivo methods to study GI motility in experimental animals.

1. Assessment of intestinal transit
2. Gastric motility
3. Measurement of gastrointestinal transit

4. Measurement of colon motility
5. Long term recording of intestinal mechanical and electrical activity.

## Assessment of gastric motility:

The function of the stomach includes initiation of digestion by exocrine secretions such as acid and pepsin, which are under the control of the endocrine secretion of hormones that also coordinate intestinal motility. Various techniques have been developed to assess gastric motility causing the gastric emptying (GE). The influence of drugs on gastric mechanical action on the bioavailability of novel compounds is of critical importance in drug development. Disturbed gastric my electric activity leading to gastro paresis can cause delayed GE, often found in patients with diabetics mellitus. Electro astrograph (EGG) may be used to evaluate the influence of prokinetics and other drugs on this condition and aid in determining effective therapy.

Intestinal motility is regulated by the enteric nervous system of the gut (Auerbachs and messengers plexuses) and the activity of this system can be modified by atomic nervous system. Hence effect of sympathomimetic and parasympathomimetic drugs on intestinal motility can be studied by using isolated piece of intestine. parasymimetic drugs stimulate enteric neurons to release acetylcholine at neuromuscular junctions and enhance muscle tone and rhythm city. Many animal models can be employed to study intestinal motility of sympathetic and parasympathetic drugs. Guinea pig ileum is advantageous for assay purpose as it produces steady baseline for studying effects of drugs. Rabbit intestine (ileum, duodenum, jejunum) usually jejunum is used for the effects of pendulum movements (continuous contraction and relaxation – Finke man method). In the present study rabbit ileum is selected for estimating the effects of selected drugs on intestinal motility.

## Requirements:

**Animals:** Medium sized rabbit

**Drugs:** Adrenaline/ Acetylcholine – 10ug/ml, Atropine Sulphate – 10ug/ ml, isoproterenol/ isopernaline 10ug/ml, Propranolol – 10mg/ml,

**Solutions:** Tyrone solution

**Apparatus used:** Kymograph, Dissecting board, Dissecting instruments, scissors, petriplates, syringe, Frontal writing lever, water bath with temperature controlling unit, organ bath with aeration tube.

## Procedure:

1. Select a medium sized rabbit for the study.
2. Fast the animal for 24 hours prior to experiment as food in gut results in messy dissection and flushing or gut contents may damage the intestine.
3. Before sacrificing the rabbit, prepare Thyroids Ringer solution and place about 250ml of this solution in an ice cold flask.
4. Sacrifice the animal by cervical decapitation without use of anesthetic as it may affect the gut motility. Shave the abdomen of the animal and vacuum the surface to remove adhered fur. Make a midline incision through the skin and abdominal muscles.
5. Locate ileum and a part of ileum was taken 10cm away from ileocaecal value.
6. An optimal length of tissue (5-6cms) is cut carefully and tie the thread to and mesenteric border on both sides and place them in Thyroid solution (extra pieces of ileum can be stored in ice cold Thyroid solution so that they are viable for hours. In ice cold solution the motility will ceases but after placing them in warm solution the tissue gets relaxed and shows motility within 5-10 minutes).
7. Record the rhythmic activity of the ileum by using frontal writing lever and kymograph. Suspend the tissue in organ bath of Thyroid solution (100ml) at 37c with adequate oxygen supply (mixture of 95% O and 5% of Co).
8. Tie one end of the thread of tissue of fixed point inside the organ bath and the other end to the lever for recording constructions on the kymograph. Stabilize the tissue in the solution to the conditions for about 30 minutes.
9. Ensure the lever should be placed horizontally and record the normal constructions followed by effects of drugs on muscles. After recording normal constructions inject the drugs one by one and observe for force of contraction and tone (normal, increased or decreased), frequency of constructions (per minute) before and after drug administration. Inject 0.1ml of drugs in the succession order in the organ bath and the responses are recorded.
10. After nothing the effect of every drug, drain the muscle bath and refill with fresh warm tyroid solution (100ml). Take the control (without drug) reading before and after each drug response.
11. Maintain washout period for 15-20 minutes for change of every drug and check the next drug response only the when the tone and amplitude returned to original value approximately.
12. The drug and dose name should be mentioned in the recording after taking response of each drug.

## Conclusion:

The effect of drugs on intestinal motility can be easily interpreted by the responses taken on kymograph.

## Precautions:

1. For experiment animal should be fasted 24 hours.
2. Care to be taken during dissection.
3. Prepare fresh physiological salt solution
4. Drug should be added in order

## VIVA-VOCE

**Q.1 Define gastrointestinal motility.**

**Ans:** Gastrointestinal motility refers to the movement of food from the mouth through the pharynx, esophagus, stomach, small and large intestines and out of the body.

**Q.2 What is motility.**

**Ans:** Motility is a term used to describe the contraction of the muscles that mix and propel contents in the gastrointestinal tract.

**Q.3 What is Achalasia.**

**Ans:** Achalasia is an esophageal motility disorder. It is diagnosed when there is a complete lack of peristalsis within the body of the esophagus. The lower esophageal sphincter does not relax to allow food to enter the stomach.

# Experiment No. 6

## Object: To study the effect of agonist and antagonists on guinea pig ileum.

## Theory:

Guinea pig ileum is a smooth muscle receive dual nerve supply from autonomic nervous system (sympathetic and parasympathetic).Parasympathetic tone is dominant in ileum which Ach cause contraction by stimulating M3-R.

## Types of receptors present in guinea-pig ileum:

- Cholinergic receptors
- Serotonergic or tryptaminergic receptors (5-HT1$\rightarrow$5-HT7)
- Histaminergic receptors
- Adrenergic receptors

Stimulation of presynaptic alpha-adrenoceptors has been shown to reduce the release of noradrenaline from postganglionic sympathetic nerve endings. Presynaptic alpha adrenoceptors located on the endings of postganglionic sympathetic fibres are dissimilar from classical postsynaptic alpha-adrenoceptors whereas phenylephrine and methoxamine act preferentially on postsynaptic ones. Some alpha adrenoceptor blocking agents such as phentolamine, yohimbine and piperoxan antagonize more readily the effects of clonidine on presynaptic alpha-adrenoceptors. In contrast, prazosin is a preferentially postsynaptic alpha-adrenoceptor blocking agent and antagonizes the effects of alpha-sympathomimetic agent such as phenylephrine and methoxamine on postsynaptic adrenoceptors.

## Requirements:

**Animal:** Guinea-pigs of either sex weighing 300-350 gm

**Drug and chemicals:** Tyrode's solution (Composition: NaC1 8g, KCI 0.2g, $CaCl_2$ 0.2g, $MgC1_2$ 0.1g, $NaH_2PO_4$ 0.05 g, glucose 0.5 g, $NaHCO_3$ 1 g for 1 L of distilled water)

## Procedure:

1. Guinea-pigs of either sex weighing 300-350 g were killed by a blow on the head and bled from the carotid arteries. 3 or 4 segments of 1.5-2 cm were removed from the terminal part of the ileum 6 to 12 cm above the ileocaecal junction.

2. The strips were placed in a 20 ml organ bath in tyrode solution. This medium was maintained at 370$^0$ C and bubbled with a constant stream of 5 % $CO_2$ in $O_2$.
3. Coaxial stimulation of the guinea-pig ileum was performed with a neuro-stimulator by means of two platinum electrodes, one placed in the lumen of the ileum and the other in the bath. The ileum preparation was equilibrated for at least 1 h before the experiments started.
4. Supramaximal current (duration I ms, frequency 5Hz, supramaximal voltage from 4 to 10V) was applied during a 5 s period every 30 s (without drug or 30 s after addition of drugs to the bath).
5. The contractions were recorded on a smoked drum by means of an isotonic lever. An initial load of 2 g was applied to the preparation.
6. Drugs were added to the bath after contractions elicited by electrical stimulation had become constant.

## Precautions:

1. Prepare tyrode's solution carefully.
2. Carefully remove ileum of guinea pigs
3. Provide constant supply of CO2
4. Drug should be added very carefully with exact concentration

## VIVA-VOCE

**Q.1 Define agonist.**

**Ans:** An agonist is a chemical that activates a receptor to produce a biological response

**Q.2 Define antagonist.**

**Ans:** An antagonist is a drug that blocks receptors without activating them.

# Experiment No. 7

## Object: To study the estimation of serum biochemical parameters by using semi-autoanalyser.

## Theory:

Serum biochemistry refers to the chemical analysis of blood serum. A profile of tests can be combined to evaluate renal function, electrolyte metabolism, serum proteins, digestion, injury, lipids, pancreatic function, and the liver.

## Serum biochemistry-

Serum biochemistry refers to the chemical analysis of serum. There are many substances in serum, including proteins, enzymes, lipids, hormones etc. Testing for these various substances provides information about the organs and tissues in the body as well as the metabolic state of the animal. If a test result is abnormal, it may indicate that disease is present. Further assessment of the test results may offer clues about which organ system is affected and also the nature and severity of the disorder.

**Renal function-** blood urea nitrogen (BUN) and creatinine.

**Electrolytes-** chloride, potassium, phosphorus, calcium, magnesium.

**Liver-** alanine aminotransferase (ALT), aspartate aminotransterase (AST),alkaline phosphatase, gamma-glutamyltransferase (GGT), total and direct bilirubin, albumin.

**Pancreas-** amylase, lipase, glucose

**Serum proteins-** total protein, albumin, globulin

**Injury-**creatine kinase (CK), lactate dehydrogenase (LDH)

**Lipids-**cholesterol, triglycerides, high-density lipoprotein (HDL), low-density lipoprotein (LDL), very low-density protein (VLDL).

**Serum Biochemical Parameters-** The two main types of protein found in blood are called albumin and globulin. These proteins can be measured individually, or combined into a single test called total protein, which measures all protein in the sample. Albumin levels can indicate if a patient is dehydrated, and can provide information about the function of the liver, kidneys, and digestive system. Globulin levels reflect underlying inflammation and/or antibody production. Increased levels of globulins are often associated with infectious diseases, immune-mediated disease, and some types of cancer.

**Liver Enzymes-** There are many different liver enzymes, but the two that appear in most profiles are alanine aminotransferase (ALT), and alkaline phosphatase (ALP). The first enzyme is typically found when the cells of the liver are stressed or damaged. The second enzyme is generally increased when bile flow in the liver is reduced.

Bilirubin is a pigment produced primarily in the liver that is associated with the breakdown of hemoglobin from red blood cells. Bilirubin is stored in the gall bladder as a component of bile. Increases in bilirubin are associated with increased red cell destruction or decreased bile through the liver.

**Kidney tests (urea, creatinine)-** The two substances most commonly measured to assess kidney function are urea (also called blood urea nitrogen or BUN) and creatinine. Urea is a by-product of protein breakdown; it is produced in the liver and excreted from the body by the kidney. Increases in BUN may indicate dehydration, gastrointestinal bleeding, cardiac disease, or primary kidney disease. Decreases in BUN are associated with over hydration liver failure or reduced protein intake in the diet. Creatinine is a by-product of muscle metabolism and it is excreted entirely by the kidney. Increased levels of creatinine indicate decreased kidney function.

**Pancreatic Enzymes (amylase, lipase, PLD)-** Two commonly measured pancreatic enzymes are amylase and lipase. Increases in these enzymes may occur when the pancreas is inflamed, although they can also be elevated with kidney or intestinal disease, and when certain drugs are used. They are not very reliable indicators of pancreatitis. A newer test for pancreatic inflammation called pancreatic lipase immunoreactivity (PLID is more reliable because it rises only with pancreatic inflammation (see handouts Pancreatitis in Cats Pancreas-Specific Lipase and Pancreatitis in Dogs - Pancreas-Specific Lipase").

**Calcium and Phosphorus-** These minerals are present in tiny amounts in blood, and changes, either up or down, may be associated with a variety of diseases or conditions. For example persistently high calcium levels may indicate the presence of kidney disease, cancer, or disease of the parathyroid glands, while low calcium levels may be due to pancreatitis, antifreeze poisoning, or disease of the parathyroid gland. High phosphorus levels are associate with kidney failure and some nutritional problems. Low phosphorous level can occur with dietary problems, gastrointestinal disease, and kidney disease etc.

**Muscle Enzymes (CK, AST, ALT)-** Creatinine kinase (CK) is the enzyme most frequently measured to assess injury of lesser importance are the enzymes aspartate aminotransferase (AST) and alanine aminotransferase (ALT), which are also used to asses liver function. Increased muscle enzyme levels are often found with muscular activity (exercise, exertion, convulsions etc) as well as trauma and muscle inflammation.

**Cholesterol-** is produced in the liver as part of fat metabolism. Increases in cholesterol are associated with hormonal and metabolic diseases, liver disease, and serious kidney disease.

**Electrolytes-** The most important electrolytes are potassium, chloride, sodium, bicarbonate. These substances are present in blood in small quantities, and each electrolvte has a different role to play in the body. Collectively, electrolytes help to maintain blood and tissue fluids in balanced state. Disturbances in electrolytes are often caused by vomiting, diarrhea, and kidney disease, and accompany many serious metabolic disorder.

## Estimation of total bilirubin:

### Principle:

Bilirubin reacts with diazotized sulphonilic acid to convert into colored compound of azobilirubin. The unconjugated bilirubin reacts with sulphonilic acid in the presence of caffine-benzoate accelerator. The colour intensity formed is directly proportional to the content of bilirubin present in the sample.

### Requirements:

**Chemical:** Bilirubin reagent, Total nitrite reagent.

**Apparatus:** Incubator, Autoanalyzer

### Procedure:

1. Total bilirubin content was measured according to manufactures protocol provided in biochemical kit.
2. Total bilirubin reagent (1 ml) mixed with total nitrite reagent (0.05 ml) and 0.1 ml sample was added in mixture and incubated for 10 minutes at room temperature.
3. The absorbance was taken at 546 nm by end point method by autoanalyzer.

### Calculation:

Total bilirubin = Absorbance of test * 13

### Precautions:

1. Care should be taken during collection of blood.
2. Carefully collect serum from blood.
3. Carefully take accurate quantity of serum to estimate biochemical parameters.
4. Calibrate auto-analyzer before stating the experiment.

# VIVA-VOCE

**Q.1 Define serum biochemistry.**

**Ans:** Serum biochemistry refers to the chemical analysis of serum. There are many substances in serum, including proteins, enzymes, lipids, hormones etc. Testing for these various substances provides information about the organs and tissues in the body as well as the metabolic state of the animal. If a test result is abnormal, it may indicate that disease is present. Further assessment of the test results may offer clues about which organ system is affected and also the nature and severity of the disorder.

**Q.2 What is principle in estimation of serum bilirubin.**

**Ans:** Bilirubin reacts with diazotized sulphonilic acid to convert into colored compound of azobilirubin. The unconjugated bilirubin reacts with sulphonilic acid in the presence of caffine-benzoate accelerator. The colour intensity formed is directly proportional to the content of bilirubin present in the sample.

**Q.3 Give the role of cholesterol.**

**Ans:** Cholesterol is produced in the liver as part of fat metabolism. Increases in cholesterol are associated with hormonal and metabolic diseases, liver disease, and serious kidney disease.

# Experiment No. 8

## Object: To study the effect of saline purgative on frog intestine.

### Theory:

Saline purgatives are the salts comprising of highly charged ions and not crosses cell membrance freely. They remain inside the lumen and retain water through osmotic forces. They increase the volume of the contents of the bowel, stretch the colon and produces normal stimulus for contraction of the muscle that leads to defecation. The aim of the present study is to examine the effect of saline purgative on frog intestine.

### Requirements:

**Animals:** frog

**Chemicals and reagents:** hypotonic solution (0.9 % to 0.45% saline), hypertonic magnesium sulphate (27%), isotonic frog's ringer solution.

**Instruments Used:** Frog's board, Pitching needle, dissecting instruments, needle with thread, and tuberculin syringe with needle.

### Procedure:

1. First immobilize the frog and place on dissecting board.
2. Expose the abdominal cavity and carefully trace the small intestine.
3. Make the small intestine into three compartments by tying threads of different colors in such a way that no fluid can move from one compartments to other compartments.
4. Then inject 0.2 ml of hypotonic solution in first compartment.
5. Inject 0.2 ml hypertonic solution in second compartments.
6. Finally inject 0.2 ml isotonic solution into third compartments.
7. Wait for 20 minutes and observe the changes.

### Observation table:

| S.No | Drug | Compartment | Observation/effect |
|---|---|---|---|
| 1. | Hypotonic solution(0.9% to 0.45% saline) | First | Shrinkage |
| 2. | Hypertonic magnesium sulphate (27%) | Second | Swollen |
| 3. | Isotonic frog's ringer solution | Third | No change |

## Conclusion:

1. In first compartment due to hypotonic solution movement of fluid occurs from lumen into circulation through process of osmosis and causes shrinkage of tissue.
2. In second compartment due to hypertonic solution movement of fluid occurs from cell into lumens and causes swelling of tissue.
3. In case of isotonic solution they don't shows any fluid movements.

## Precautions:

1. Immobilize frog carefully
2. Use sterile surgical
3. Carefully expose abdominal cavity
4. Clean all apparatus and glassware before stating the experiment
5. Prepare carefully hypotonic and hypertonic solution

## VIVA-VOCE

**Q.1 Define saline purgatives.**

**Ans:** Saline purgatives are the salts comprising of highly charged ions and not crosses cell membrance freely. They remain inside the lumen and retain water through osmotic forces. They increase the volume of the contents of the bowel, stretch the colon and produces normal stimulus for contraction of the muscle that leads to defecation.

**Q.2 Define hypotonic solution.**

**Ans:** A hypotonic solution is any solution that has a lower osmotic pressure than another solution.

**Q.3 Define hypertonic solution.**

**Ans:** A hypertonic solution contains a higher concentration of solutes compared to another solution.

**Q.4 Define isotonic solution.**

**Ans:** An isotonic solution refers to two solution having the same osmotic pressure across a semipermeable membrane.

# Experiment No. 9

## Object: To study the insulin hypoglycemic effect in rabbit.

## Theory:

Diabetes mellitus, a metabolic disorder, is characterized by hyperglycemia, altered metabolism of lipids, carbohydrates and proteins with an increased risk of complications of vascular diseases. Diabetes may be insulin dependent (IDDM) or non-insulin dependent (NIDDM). In insulin dependent diabetes mellitus also known as type 1 diabetes mellitus, the beta cells of islets of langerhans of pancreas of the patients are either malfunctioning or destroyed. The NIDDM or type 2 diabetes mellitus is the most prevalent form of the disease. The type 2 diabetes patient exhibit insulin resistance and ultimately develop concomitant insulin secretory defect.

Insulin is a hormone made by the pancreas that allows your body to use sugar (glucose) from carbohydrates in the food that you eat for energy or to store glucose for future use. Insuline helps keeps your blood sugar level from getting too high (hyperglycemia) or too low (hypoglycemia).

## Insulin treatment for diabetes:

People with type 1 diabetes cannot make insulin because the beta cells in their pancreas are damaged or destroyed. Therefore, these people will need insulin injections to allow their body to process glucose and avoid complications from hyperglycemia.

Various types of insulin are used to treat diabetes and include:

**Rapid-acting insulin:** It starts working approximately 15 minutes after injection and peaks at approximately 1 hour but continues to work for two to four hours. This is usually taken before a meal and in addition to a long acting insulin.

**Short acting insulin:** It starts working approximately 30 minutes after injection and peaks at approximately 2 to 3 hours but will continue to work for three to six hours. It is usually given before a meal and in addition to a long acting insulin.

**Intermediate acting insulin:** It starts working approximately 2 to 4 hour after injection and peaks at approximately 4 to 12 hours later and continues to work for 12 to 18 hours. It is usually taken twice a day and in addition to a rapid or short acting insulin.

**Long acting insulin:** It starts working after several hours after injection and works for approximately 24 hours. If necessary, it is often used in combination with rapid or short acting insulin.

## Requirements:

**Animals:** Rabbits weighing between 2.0-3.0 kg

**Chemicals and Drugs:** insulin preparation, normal saline, HCL, 15% glycerin, 0.5 % phenol

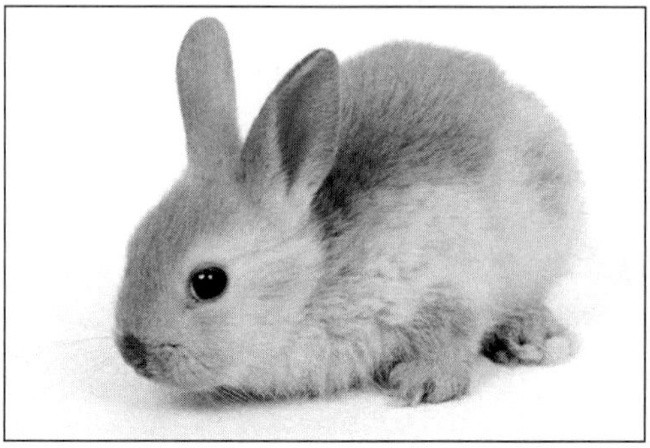

**Rabbit**

## Procedure:

1. Take healthy rabbit weighing between 2.0- 3.0 kg.
2. They should be provided with free access of diet and water for 7 days.
3. Kept animals at fasting at least 12 hours before starting the experiments.
4. Select at least 3 animals for study and inject 1 unit/ml of insulin.
5. Prepare drug solution freshly.
6. Weigh 20 units of insulin accurately and dissolve it in normal saline.
7. Acidify the solution by using HCL to pH 2.5.
8. Add 0.5 % of phenol as a preservative and 1.5 % glycerine and make the final volume to 20 units/ml of solution.
9. Withdraw 2 ml blood from marginal ear vein of each rabbit and estimate blood glucose level by using suitable biochemical methods and the concentration of glucose can be noted as initial blood glucose level.
10. Then inject insulin 1 unit/ml to the animals and check blood glucose level up to 5 hrs at interval of 1 hr.
11. Finally determine the blood glucose level by comparing initial and final blood glucose level.

## Observation table:

| S.No. | Animal no. | Initial blood glucose level (mg/ml) | Final blood glucose level in time intervals of hours (mg/ml) | | | | |
|---|---|---|---|---|---|---|---|
| | | | 1 | 2 | 3 | 4 | 5 |
| 1. | 1 | | | | | | |
| 2. | 2 | | | | | | |
| 3. | 3 | | | | | | |
| Average value | | | | | | | |

**Conclusion:** Percentage decrease in blood glucose level determines the effect of insulin.

## Precautions:

1. Handle the animal carefully during experiment.
2. Prepare drug solution freshly before stating the experiment.
3. Take the accurate weight of animals.
4. Inject the accurate volume of drug in animals.
5. Care to be taken during withdrawal of blood from animals.
6. Care should be taken during of blood glucose level estimation by using suitable biochemical kit.

## VIVA-VOCE

**Q.1 Explain in details about insulin.**

**Ans:** Insuline is a chemical messenger that allows cells to absorb glucose from the blood. The pancrease is an organ behind the stomach that is the main source of insulin in the body. Clusters of cells in the pancreas called islets produce the hormone and determine the amount based on blood glucose levels in the body.

**Q.2 What is mean by hyperglycemia.**

**Ans:** It is a condition in which an excessive amount of sugar circulates in the blood plasma.

**Q.3 What is mean by hypoglycemia.**

**Ans:** Hypoglycemia is a condition caused by a very low level of blood sugar.

**Q.4 Explain the role of HCL and Phenol in experiment.**

**Ans:** HCL used to acidify the solution and phenol is used as preservative for solutions.

# Experiment No. 10

## Object: To study the test for pyrogens (rabbit method).

## Theory:

**Pyrogen:** These are the agents that cause rise in temperature which can be polysaccharide or protein in nature.

Typically, pyrogenic substances include endotoxin and other bacterial byproducts. The typical assay for endotoxin contamination detection is the LAL test. In some cases, the LAL may not be feasible. The rabbit pyrogen test, in addition to the LAL test, as an alternative assay for the detection of endotoxin and other pyrogens. The rabbit pyrogen test requires the injection of a small amount of batched test material into a rabbits blood stream, and monitoring for temperature increases.

The pyrogen test is aim to check the existence of pyrogen by using rabbits. The pyrogen test is based on the measurement of the increase in the rabbits body temperature by injecting the product that might contain a contaminant of the pyrogen type. The Pyrogen is the substance that causes an increase in fever called as pyrexia.

Treatment with antipyretics has been very important in the pre-antibiotic era. So that, treatment for acute viral diseases and treatment of protozoal infections like malaria there is reduction in elevated body temperature by using antipyretics. As to evaluate these properties of antipyretics fever is induced in rabbits or rats by injection of lipopolysaccharide or brewer's yeast.

**Endotoxin:** It is a type of pyrogen and is component of outer wall of gram negative bacteria, chemically it is lipopolysaccharide.

## Requirements:

**Animals:** Healthy rabbit (not less than 1.5 kg)

**Chemicals and Drugs:** Test solution

**Instruments and apparatus:** thermometer, syringe and injection needle.

## Procedure:

1. Place the animal in experiment room its environment is similar to animal housed room.
2. Remove the feed and water before starting the experiment.

3. The test animal fix in suitable holder.
4. Make syringe and injecting needles pyrogens free by heating at $250^0$ C for 30 minutes.
5. Insert the thermometer in rectum of animal in constant depth of 60-90 mm and record temperature for sufficient time period.
6. Determine temperature 3 times of interval of 1 hours before injection of sample.
7. If 2nd and 3rd temperature has little difference them latter taken as control temperature. Do not use animals whose 2nd and 3rd temperature are not in accord.
8. Warm the sample at $37^0$ C before injection, and administer intravenously in ear vein within 15 minutes after 3rd temperature recording.
9. Read the temperature 3 times of 1 hour interval after sample injection
10. The difference between control temperature and highest temperature is taken for rise in temperature.

## Observation table:

| Number of rabbits | Initial body temperature (°C) | | | Final body temperature (°C) | | |
|---|---|---|---|---|---|---|
| | 60 Min | 120 Min | 180 Min | 60 Min | 120 Min | 180 Min |
| 1 | | | | | | |
| 2 | | | | | | |
| 3 | | | | | | |

## Precautions:

1. Prepare test solution as per guidelines.
2. All apparatus and instruments should be sterilized before experiment.
3. Animal should be kept carefully in animal holder.
4. Carefully inject test substance in animals.
5. Calibrate thermometer before use in experiment.

## VIVA-VOCE

**Q.1 What is mean by pyrogen.**

**Ans:** A pyrogen is a substance causing rise in temperature which can be polysaccharide or protein in nature. Typically, pyrogenic substances include endotoxin and other bacterial byproducts.

**Q.2 What is endotoxin.**

**Ans:** Endotoxin is a type of pyrogen and is component of outer wall of gram negative bacteria, chemically it is lipopolysaccharide.

**Q.3 What is LAL test.**

**Ans:** The LAL test is a test for the determination of bacterial endotoxins, which uses an Amobocyte Lysate of the Limulus crab. In this test, the reactions which occur in the Amobocyte Lysate as a result of a defence mechanism of the crab in the presence of endotoxins and which conclude with a gelation process are used. These occur when a chromophore is added to the environment so that a colour changes is achieved related to the reactions triggered by the endotoxins.

**Q.4 Why the rabbit in pyrogen test.**

**Ans:** Rabbits are used in pyrogen test because

i. Reproducible pyrogenic response
ii. Other species not predictable
iii. Similar threshold pyrogenic response to humans
iv. Rabbit chosen for economic purposes.

# Experiment No. 11

## Object: To study the determination of acute oral toxicity ($LD_{50}$) of a drug from a given data.

## Theory:

Acute systemic toxicity evaluates the adverse effects that occur following exposure of organisms to a single or multiple doses of a test substance within 24 hours by a known route (oral, dermal or inhalation). After administration, the test substance is absorbed and distributed to various parts of the body before it elicits systemic adverse effect. The regulatory body requires the acute toxicity test report for labeling and classification of substances for human use. The $LD_{50}$ (median lethal dose) test was introduced in 1927 by J.W Trevan to estimate the dose of a test substance that produces 50% death in a given species of animals. It is usually the first conducted for every chemical before further toxicity tests are carried out. It is used for estimating the potential hazards of chemicals on humans. Although its major endpoint is death, non-lethal acute effect may occur as signs of toxicity depending on the chemical being tested. Assessment of the acute toxic potential of substances is required to determine their adverse effects that might occur due to accidental or deliberate short-term toxicity studies as well as other studies that involve the use of animals. From the result of an acute toxicity test, a conclusion can be made on the toxicity status of the test substance.

## The conventional $LD_{50}$ test:

This is the first acute toxicity test that was developed in the $1920_s$. It was called "Classical $LD_{50}$" Where large numbers of animals, up to 100 animals for five dose-groups is used. Animal are dosed with the test chemical to determine the dose that would result in 50 percent deaths.

## 1931 Karbal method:

This method was introduced in 1931 and it involves the use of 30 animals which are divided into six groups of five animals each. The animals are dosed with the test substance and observed for the first four hours, 24 hours and daily for 14-days for signs of toxicity. At the end of 14 days the total number of death is recorded. The sum of the product of dose difference and mean death is divided by the number of animals in each group and the resulting quotient is subtracted from the non-lethal dose to obtain the $LD_{50}$ value.

$$LD_{50} = LD_{100} - \{\Sigma[\text{Dose difference x Mean dead}]\}/\text{Number of animals per group}$$

## 1938 Arithmetical Method of Reed and Muench:

After the conventional $LD_{50}$ test, the Arithmetical Method of Reed and Muench was introduced in 1938. In this test, animals are expose to the chemical and the log dose, number of death and survival, cumulative death and survival are calculated. These are used for $LD_{50}$ determination. However, in 2011, a modification which involved calculation of test animals that die and survive was made by saganuwan. In this approach, forty test animals were divided into four groups of 10 animals each.

## 1940: Approximate lethal dose:

Due to the limitations characterized by high mortality rate in the conventional $LD_{50}$ test, an alternative procedure for the determination of approximate lethal dose was developed in the early $1940_{s.}$ The animals are administered with the dose of the test substance that increases by 50 percent over the previous dose.

## 1944: Miller and Tainter method:

The Miller and Tainter method was established in 1944. It involves the use of fifty animals which are divided into five groups of ten animals each. Signs of toxicity and death are observed and recorded after administration and the $LD_{50}$ is calculated using probit analysis table. Probit values are plotted against log doses and the dose corresponding to probit five becomes the $LD_{50}$ value.

## Calculation of $LD_{50}$ tests according to OECD guideline:

In 1981, the Organization for Economic Cooperation and Development (OECD) incorporated the $LD_{50}$ test into its new test guidelines. It involves the use of 30 animals for 3 doses. In 1987 the OECD further modified this method by reducing the number from 30 to 20 animals where five animals per dose level are selected based on sighting studies or from historical data of the chemical to be tested.

An upper dose level limit of 5,000 mg/kg was also introduced essentially for substances whose $LD_{50}$ values exceed 5.000 mg/kg. Similar guidelines were also published for acute dermal and inhalation toxicity. The limit test is usually employed whenever a test substance is suspected to be non-toxic based on historical information about the test substance. In this regard, determination of the precise $LD_{50}$ would not be necessary, but the limit test can be employed. This involves the exposure of few number of animals to large dose (5,000mg/kg) of the test chemical. If animals survive, the $LD_{50}$ is estimated to be above 5000 mg/kg and no further acute toxicity testing is required.

# VIVA-VOCE

**Q.1 What is mean by $LD_{50}$**

**Ans:** The name $LD_{50}$ is an abbreviation for "Lethal Dose, 50%" or median lethal dose. It is the amount of the substances required (usually per body weight) to kill 50% of the test population.

**Q.2 Enlist conventional methods for estimation of $LD_{50}$.**

**Ans:** Following are some conventional methods for estimation of $LD_{50}$

i. Karbal method
ii. Arithmetical method of Reed and Muench
iii. Approximate lethal dose
iv. Miller and Tainter method

**Q.3 What is full form of OECD guidelines.**

**Ans:** Full form of OECD is Organization for Economic Cooperation and Development.

**Q.4 The role of the $LD_{50}$ determination in drug safety evaluation.**

**Ans:** Acute toxicological studies in animals are essential to drug development. Often such experiments seek to establish precisely the median lethal dose ($LD_{50}$) in rodents. As scientific needs rarely require an exact value, practices and regulations should be changed to provide the option of obtaining adequate information on the acute toxicity of a drug with fewer animals than the precise $LD_{50}$ test demands.

# Experiment No. 12

## Object: To study the determination of acute skin irritation/corrosion of a test substance.

### Theory:

Dermal irritation is the production of reversible damage of the skin following the application of a test substance for up to 4 hours.

Dermal corrosion is the production of irreversible damage of the skin; namely, visible necrosis through the epidermis and into the dermis, following the application of a test substance for up to four hours. Corrosive reactions are typified by ulcers, bleeding, bloody scabs, and by the end of observation at 14 days, by discolouration due to blanching of the skin, complete areas of alopecia, and scars. Histopathology should be considered to evaluate questionable lesions.

In the interest of both sound science and animal welfare, in vivo testing should not be undertaken until all available data relevant to the potential dermal corrosivity/irritation of the substance have been evaluated in a weight of the evidence analysis. Such data will include evidence from existing studies in humans and/or laboratory animals, avidence of corrosivity/irritation of one or more structurally related substances or mixtures of such substances, data demonstrating strong acidity or alkalinity of the substance, and results from validated and accepted in vitro or ex vivo tests. This analysis should decrease the need for in vivo testing for dermal corrosovoty/irritation of substances for which sufficient evidence already exists from other studies as to those two endpoints.

### Principle:

The test chemical to be tested is applied in a single dose to the skin of an experimental animal, untreated skin areas of the test animal serve as the control. The degree of irritation/ corrosion is read and scored as specified intervals. Animals showing continuening signs of serve distress and/or pain at any stage of the test should be humanely killed, and the test chemical assessed accordingly.

### Procedure:

As per OECD guidelines no 404

## Preparations for the in vivo test:

### Selection of animal species:

The albino rabbit is the preferable laboratory animal, and healthy young adult rabbits are used. A rationale for using other species should be provided.

### Preparation of the animals:

Approximately 24 hours before the test, fur should be removed by closely clipping the dorsal area of the trunk of the animals. Care should be taken to avoid abrading the skin, and only animals with healthy, intact skin should be used. Some strains of rabbit have dense patches of hair that are more prominent at certain times of the year. Such areas of dense hair growth should not be used as test sites.

### Housing and feeding conditions:

Animals should be individually housed. The temperature of the experimental animal room should be 20°C (± 3°C) for rabbits. Although the relative humidity should be at least 30% and preferably not exceed 70%, other than during room cleaning, the aim should be 50-60%. Lighting should be artificial, the sequence being 12 hours light, 12 hours dark. For feeding, conventional laboratory diets may be used with an unrestricted supply of drinking water.

## Test procedure:

### Application of the test substance:

The test substance should be applied to a small area (approximately 6 cm) of skin and covered with a gauze patch, which is held in place with non-irritating tape. In cases in which direct application is not possible (e.g., liquids or some pastes), the test substance should first be applied to the gauze patch, which is then applied to the skin. The patch should be loosely held in contact with the skin by means of a suitable semi-occlusive dressing for the duration of the exposure period. If the test substance is applied to the patch, it should be attached to the skin in such a manner that there is good contact and uniform distribution of the substance on the skin. Access by the animal to the patch and ingestion or inhalation of the test substance should be prevented.

Liquid test substances are generally used undiluted. When testing solids (which may be pulverized, if considered necessary), the test substance should be moistened with the smallest amount of water (or, where necessary, of another suitable vehicle) sufficient to ensure good skin contact. When vehicles other than water are used, the potential influence of the vehicle on irritation of the skin by the test substance should be minimal, if any.

At the end of the exposure period, which is normally 4 hours, residual test substance should be removed, where practicable, using water or an appropriate solvent without altering the existing response or the integrity of the epidermis.

## Dose level:

A dose of 0.5 ml of liquid or 0.5 gm of solid or paste is applied to the test site.

**Initial test:** (in vivo dermal irritation/corrosion test using one animal)

It is strongly recommended that the in vivo test be performed initially using one animal, especially when the substance is suspected to have corrosion potential. This is in accordance with the sequential testing strategy (Supplement).

When a substance has been judged to be corrosive on the basis of a weight-of-the-evidence analysis, no further animal testing is needed. For most substances suspected of being corrosive, further in vivo testing is normally not necessary. However, in those cases where additional data are felt warranted because of insufficient evidence, limited animal testing may be carried out using the following approach:

Up to three test patches are applied sequentially to the animal. The first patch is removed after three minutes. If no serious skin reaction is observed, a second patch is applied at a different site and removed after one hour. If the observations at this stage indicate that exposure can humanely be allowed to extend to four hours, a third patch is applied and removed after four hours, and the response is graded.

If a corrosive effect is observed after any of the three sequential exposures, the test is immediately terminated. If a corrosive effect is not observed after the last patch is removed the animal is observed for 14 days, unless corrosion develops at an earlier time point.

In those cases in which the test substance is not expected to produce corrosion but may be irritating, a single patch should be applied to one animal for four hours.

**Confirmatory test**: (in vivo dermal irritation test with additional animals)

If a corrosive effect is not observed in the initial test, the irritant or negative response should be confirmed using up to two additional animals, each with one patch, for an exposure period of four hours.

If an irritant effect is observed in the initial test, the confirmatory test may be conducted in a sequential manner, or by exposing two additional animals simultaneously. In the exceptional case, in which the initial test is not conducted, two or three animals may be treated with a single patch, which is removed after four hours. When two animals are used, if both exhibit the same response, no further testing is needed.

Otherwise, the third animal is also tested. Equivocal responses may need to be evaluated using additional animals.

### Observation period:

The duration of the observation period should be sufficient to evaluate fully the reversibility of the effects observed. However, the experiment should be terminated at any time that the animal shows continuing signs of severe pain or distress. To determine the reversibility of effects, the animals should be observed up to 14 days after removal of the patches. If reversibility is seen before 14 days, the experiment should be terminated at that time.

### Clinical observations and grading of skin reactions:

All animals should be examined for signs of erythema and oedema, and the response scored at 60 minutes, and then at 24, 48 and 72 hours after patch removal. For the initial test in one animal, the test site is also examined immediately after the patch has been removed.

Dermal reactions are graded and recorded according to the grades in the Table below. If there is damage to skin which cannot be identified as irritation or corrosion at 72 hours, observations may be needed until day 14 to determine the reversibility of the effects. In addition to the observation of irritation, all local toxic effects, such as defatting of the skin, and any systemic adverse effects (e.g., effects on clinical signs of toxicity and body weight), should be fully described and recorded. Histopathological examination should be considered to clarify equivocal responses.

The grading, of skin responses is necessarily subjective. To promote harmonisation in grading of skin response and to assist testing laboratories and those involved in making and interpreting the observations, the personnel performing the observations need to be adequately trained in the scoring system used.

## Precautions:

1. The test substance should be applied to a small area.
2. Care should be taken to avoid abrading the skin.
3. Observe irritation very carefully.
4. The substance to be tested is applied in a single dose to the skin of an experimental animal.

## VIVA-VOCE

**Q.1 Define dermal irritation.**

**Ans:** It is the production of reversible damage of the skin following the application of a test substance for up to 4 hours.

**Q.2 What is mean by contact dermatitis.**

**Ans:** Contact dermatitis is a reaction that appears when the skin comes in contact with an irritant or allergen.

# Experiment No. 13

## Object: To study the determination of acute eye irritation/corrosion of a substance.

## Theory:

Eye irritation is defined as "the production of changes in the eye following the application of test substance to the anterior surface of the eye, which are fully reversible within 21 days of application". Serious eye damage (eye corrosion) is defined as "the production of tissue damage in the eye, or serious physical decay of vision, following application of a test substances to the anterior surface of the eye, which is not fully reversible within 21 days of application"

The anterior surface of the eye is covered by the cornea and the conjunctiva. The cornea is the most exposed area and, therefore, the most likely part of the eye to be involved in a chemical exposure to the eye.

Chemical injury to the cornea can result in the loss of vision. Accordingly, corneal injury in the animal test for eye irritation/corrosion accounts for about 73% of the total ocular toxicity score. For these reasons, the cornea has been the primary tissue modeled in vitro assays for accessing eye injury.

The cornea is composed of three cellular layers. The outermost layer, the corneal epithelium, is composed of 5-7 epithelial cell layers in the human cornea. The surface layers of cells are connected by tight junctions that modulate the permeation of molecules into the tissue. The stroma, beneath the corneal epithelium, is composed of keratocytes (fibroblast-like cells) interspersed in the stromal collagen matrix. A single cell layer of corneal endothelial cells forms the innermost cellular layer of the cornea. Nerve cells penetrate through the cornea into the corneal epithelium, making it one of the most highly innervated tissues in the body; these cells are readily perturbed when the corneal epithelial tight junctions are disrupted. Many mild eye irritants act by disrupting or damaging only the surface cells of the corneal epithelium, and the cornea can repair this type of damage within a short time. The stronger the eye irritant, the deeper it penetrates into the next layer of the cornea, the stroma. Very damading materials might penetrate deep enough to cause irreversible injury, including damage to the corneal endothelial cell layer, where tight junctions modulate the penetration of water and other substances from the cornea to the aqueous humor. The conjunctiva covers the remaining surface of the eye and is also important in protecting the eye from environmental insults. Injury to the conjunctiva has been assigned about 18% of the in vivo eye injury score in the Draize test but has largely been ignored in vitro assessments of chemical eye injury. Conjunctival injury may be irrelevant in moderate to severe eye injury, where the corneal effects are largely predictive of reversibility and outcome, but could be useful in assessing milder effects, especially for products used in and around the eye. For example, the conjunctiva can exhibit different mechanisms of injury than the cornea due to its different physiology. The conjunctiva contains goblet cells, which secrete the mucin layer that protects the surface of the eye, as well as immune and vascular components important in the eye irritation and ocular allergy responses.

## Eye irritation test according to OECD guidelines:

### Principle of the in vivo test:

Following pre treatment with a systemic analgesic and induction of appropriate topical anesthesia, the substance to be tested is applied in a single dose to one of the eyes of the experimental animal; the untreated eye serves as the control. The degree of eye irritation/ corrosion is evaluated by scoring lesions of conjunctiva, cornea, and iris, at specific intervals. Other effects in the eye and adverse systemic effects are also described to provide a complete evaluation of the effects. The duration of the study should be sufficient to evaluate the reversibility or irreversibility of the effects. Animals showing signs of severe distress and/ or pain at any stage of the test or lesions consistent with the humane endpoints described in this Test Guideline should be humanely killed, and the substance assessed accordingly.

### Preparations for the in vivo test:

#### Selection of species:

The albino rabbit is the preferable laboratory animal and healthy young adult animals are used. A rationale for using other strains or species should be provided.

#### Preparation of animals:

Both eyes of each experimental animal provisionally selected for testing should be examined within 24 hours before testing starts. Animals showing eye irritation, ocular defects, or pre-existing corneal injury should not be used.

#### Housing and feeding conditions:

Animals should be individually housed. The temperature of the experimental animal room should be 20°C (± 3°C) for rabbits. Although the relative humidity should be at least 30% and preferably not exceed 70%, other than during room cleaning, the aim should be 50-60%.

Lighting should be artificial, the sequence being 12 hours light, 12 hours dark. Excessive light intensity should be avoided. For feeding, conventional laboratory diets may be used with an unrestricted supply of drinking water.

## Test procedure:

### Use of topical anesthetics and systemic analgesics:

The following procedures are recommended to avoid or minimize pain and distress in ocular safety testing procedures. Alternate procedures that have been determined to provide as good or better avoidance or relief of pain and distress may be substituted.

Sixty minutes prior to test substance application (TSA), buprenorphine 0.01 mg/kg is administered by subcutaneous injection (SC) to provide a therapeutic level of systemic analgesia. Buprenorphine and other similar opiod analgesics administered systemically are not known or expected to alter ocular Responses.

Five minutes prior to TSA, one or two drops of a topical ocular anesthetic (e.g. 0.5% proparacaine hydrochloride or 0.5% tetracaine hydrochloride) are applied to each eye. In order to avoid possible interference with the study, a topical anesthetic that does not contain preservatives is recommended. The eye of each animal that is not treated with a test article, but which is treated with topical anesthetics, serves as a control. If the test substance is anticipated to cause significant pain and distress, it should not normally be tested in vivo. However, in case of doubt or where testing is necessary, consideration should be given to additional applications of the topical anesthetic at 5-minute intervals prior to TSA. Users should be aware that multiple applications of topical anesthetics could potentially cause a slight increase in the severity and/or time required for chemically-induced lesions to clear.

Eight hours after TSA, buprenorphine 0.01 mg/kg SC and meloxicam 0.5 mg/kg SC are administered to provide a continued therapeutic level of systemic analgesia. While there are no data to suggest that meloxicam has anti-inflammatory effects on the eye when administered SC once daily, meloxicam should not be administered until at least 8 hours after TSA in order to avoid any possible interference with the study.

After the initial 8-hour post-TSA treatment, buprenorphine 0.01 mg/kg SC should be administered every 12 hours, in conjunction with meloxicam 0.5 mg/kg SC every 24hours, until the ocular lesions resolve and no clinical signs of pain and distress are present. Sustained-release preparations of analgesics are available that could be considered to decrease the frequency of analgesic dosing.

"Rescue" analgesia should be given immediately after TSA if pre-emptive analgesia and topical anesthesia are inadequate. If an animal shows signs of pain and distress during the study, a "rescue" dose of buprenorphine 0.03 mg/kg SC would be given immediately and repeated as often as every 8 hours, if necessary, instead of 0.01 mg/kg SC every 12 hours.

Meloxicam 0.5 mg/kg SC would be administered every 24 hours in conjunction with the "rescue" dose of buprenorphine, but not until at least 8 hours post-TSA.

## Application of the test substance:

The test substance should be placed in the conjunctival sac of one eye of each animal after gently pulling the lower lid away from the eyeball. The lids are then gently held together for about one second in order to prevent loss of the material. The other eye, which remains untreated, serves as a control.

## Irritation:

The eyes of the test animals should not be washed for at least 24 hours following instillation of the test substance, except for solids, and in case of immediate corrosive or irritating effects. At 24 hours a washout may be used if considered appropriate.

Use of a satellite group of animals to investigate the influence of washing is not recommended unless it is scientifically justified. If a satellite group is needed, two rabbits should be used. Conditions of washing should be carefully documented, e.g., time of washing; composition and temperature of wash solution; duration, volume, and velocity of application.

## Dose level:

### (1) Testing of liquids:

For testing liquids, a dose of 0.1 ml is used. Pump sprays should not be used for instilling the substance directly into the eye. The liquid spray should be expelled and collected in a container prior to instilling 0.1 ml into the eye.

### (2) Testing of solids:

When testing solids, pastes, and particulate substances, the amount used should have a volume of 0.1 ml or a weight of not more than 100 mg. The test material should be ground to a fine dust. The volume of solid material should be measured after gently compacting it, e.g. by tapping the measuring container. If the solid test substance has not been removed from the eye of the test animal by physiological mechanisms at the first observation time point of 1 hour after treatment, the eye may be rinsed with saline or distilled water.

### (3) Testing of aerosols:

It is recommended that all pump sprays and aerosols be collected prior to instillation into the eye. The one exception is for substances in pressurised aerosol containers, which cannot be collected due to vaporisation. In such cases, the eye should be held open, and the test substance administered to the eye in a simple burst of about one second, from a distance of 10 cm directly in front of the eye. This distance may vary depending on the pressure of the spray and its contents. Care should be taken not to damage the eye from the pressure of the spray. In appropriate cases, there may be a need to evaluate the potential for "mechanical" damage to the eye from the force of the spray.

An estimate of the dose from an aerosol can be made by simulating the test as follows: the substance is sprayed on to weighing paper through an opening the size of a rabbit eye placed directly before the paper. The weight increase of the paper is used to approximate the amount sprayed into the eye. For volatile substances, the dose may be estimated by weighing a receiving container before and after removal of the test material.

## Initial test (in vivo eye irritation/corrosion test using one animal):

It is strongly recommended that the in vivo test be performed initially using one animal. Observations should allow for determination of severity and reversibility before proceeding to a confirmatory test in a second animal. The results of this test indicate the substance to be corrosive or a severe irritant to the eye using the procedure described, further testing for ocular irritancy should not be performed.

## Confirmatory test (in vivo eye irritation test with additional animals):

If a corrosive or severe irritant effect is not observed in the initial test, the irritant or negative response should be confirmed using up to two additional animals. If an irritant effect is observed in the initial test, it is recommended that the confirmatory test be conducted in a sequential manner in one animal at a time, rather than exposing the two additional animals simultaneously. If the second animal reveals corrosive or severe irritant effects, the test is not continued. If results from the second animal are sufficient to allow for a hazard classification determination, then no further testing should be conducted.

## Observation period:

The duration of the observation period should be sufficient to evaluate fully the magnitude and reversibility of the effects observed. However, the experiment should be terminated at any time that the animal shows signs of severe pain or distress. To determine reversibility of effects, the animals should be observed normally for 21 days post administration of the test substance. If reversibility is seen before 21 days, the experiment should be terminated at that time.

## VIVA-VOCE

**Q.1 Define eye irritation.**

**Ans:** Eye irritation is defined as "the production of changes in the eye following the application of test substance to the anterior surface of the eye, which are fully reversible within 21 days of application"

**Q.2 Define eye corrosion.**

**Ans:** Eye corrosion is defined as "the production of tissue damage in the eye, or serious physical decay of vision, following application of a test substances to the anterior surface of the eye, which is not fully reversible within 21 days of application"

**Q.3 Define eye severe irritant.**

**Ans:** A substance that causes tissue damage in the eye that does not resolve within 21 days of application or causes serious physical decay of vision.

# Experiment No. 14

## Object: Calculation of pharmacokinetic parameters from a given data.

## Introduction:

Pharmacokinetics is currently defined as the study of the time course of drug absorption, distribution, metabolism, and excretion. Pharmacokinetics is often studied in conjunction with pharmacodynamics. Pharmacodynamics explores what a drug does to the body, whereas pharmacokinetics explores what the body does to the drug.

Pharmacokinetics includes the study of the mechanisms of absorption and distribution of an administered drug, the rate at which a drug action begins and the duration of the effect, the chemical changes of the substance in the body (e.g. by enzymes) and the effects and routes of excretion of the metabolites of the drug.

Pharmacokinetics is divided into several areas which includes the extent and rate of Absorption, Distribution, Metabolism and Excretion. This is commonly referred to as the ADME scheme. However recent understanding about the drug-body interactions brought about the inclusion of new term Liberation. Now Pharmacokinetics can be better described as LADME.

**Liberations:** The process of release of drug from the formulation.

**Absorption**: It is the process of a substance entering the body.

**Distribution:** It is the dispersion or dissemination of substances throughout the fluids and tissues of the body.

**Metabolism:** It is the irreversible transformation of parent compounds into daughter metabolites.

**Excretion**: It is the elimination of the substances from the body. In rare cases, some drugs irreversibly accumulate in a tissue in the body.

## Biliary excretion and enter hepatic cycle:

**Definition:** "Irreversible transfer of drug or drug metabolites from the plasma to the bile through the hepatocytes (biliary excretion). This can be followed by intestinal reabsorption of the active drug (enterohepatic cycle)".

Drugs are transferred from the plasma into the bile through the hepatocytes. This transport is due to active secretion of drugs into the bile by means of transport systems: e.g.

the organic anion transporting polypeptides (OATPS), the P-glycoprotein transport system and the multidrug resistance-associated proteins (Mrps). The latter are important for the excretion of conjugated metabolites.

Drug in bile entern the gastrointestinal tract after storage in the gallbladder. It may then excreted from the body by the stools.

Drugs may be excreted into the bile either in a native form or after metabolism into me polar conjugates. The bile is released in the gut lumen, from which the native drug can reabsorbed. In the small intestine, the enzymes of the intestinal flora may hydrolyze the conjugated metabolites and free the active drug, which may in turn also be reabsorbed. After penetrating the intestinal mucosa, the active drug enters the portal vein, which carries it back to the liver. This cycle is called the enterohepatic cycle and may be repeated several times significantly prolonging the body exposure to the drug.

Pharmacokinetics describes how the body affects a specific drug after administration Pharmacokinetic properties of drugs may be affected by elements administration and the concentration in which the drug is administered. These may affect the absorption rate.

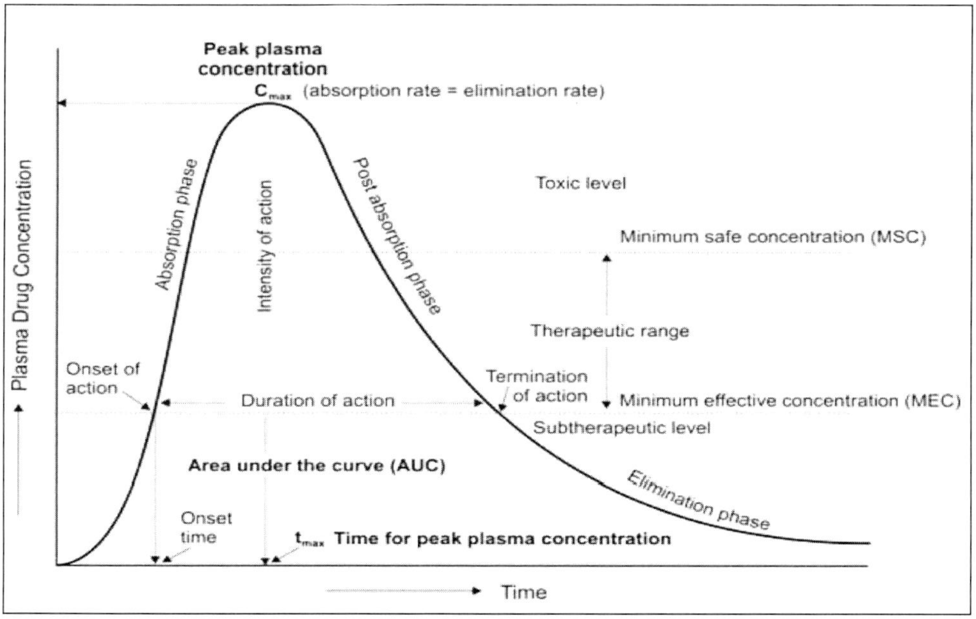


**Figure: Plasma concentration time profile**

## Biological half life (t1/2):

It is also called as elimination half life. The biological half-life or elimination half life of a substance is the time it takes for a substance (drug, radioactive nuclide, or other) to lose half of its pharmacologic, physiologic, or radiologic activity. In a medical context, half-life may also describe the time it takes for the blood plasma concentration of a substance to halve plasma half-life") of its steady-state. The relationship between the biological and plasma half-lifes of a substance can be complex, due to factors including accumulation in tissues active metabolites, and receptor interactions.

$t_{1/2} = 0.693/Ke$

Where Ke = Elimination rate constant

| S.No. | Drug | Biological half life |
|---|---|---|
| 1. | Phenytoin | 12-42 hours |
| 2. | Methadone | 15-72 hours |
| 3. | Buprenorphine | 16-72 hours |
| 4. | Clonazepam | 18-50 hours |
| 5. | Phenytoin | 12-42 hours |
| 6. | Methadone | 15-72 hours |
| 7. | Buprenorphine | 16-72 hours |
| 8. | Clonazepam | 18-50 hours |
| 9. | Flurazepam | 19-100 hours |
| 10. | Diazepam | 20-100 hours |

## Importance of biological half life:

- Adjustment of doses can be made by use of biological half life.
- Dosing regimen can be decided from biological half life.
- It is of very much importance in toxicity studies.

## Absorption rate constant:

### Introduction:

The oral absorption of drugs is often approximated assuming linear kinetics, typically when given in solution. The same is true for the absorption of drugs from many other extravascular sites, including subcutaneous tissue and muscle. Under these circumstances, absorption is characterized by an absorption rate constant and a corresponding absorption half-life.

However, the absorption of many drugs do not exactly follow linear kinetics. In some cases the drug may be absorbed at a constant rate so that the same amount of drug is absorbed during each time interval, mimicking constant rate intravenous infusion. Different factors may be responsible for nonlinear absorption such as controlled-release formulations or saturable transport mechanisms of the drug from the intestinal lumen to the portal circulation.

Expressed by Ka, The rate of drug absorption can be zero order, first order, pseudo zero order, pseudo first order, etc. Generally for I.R dosage form Ka is first order because of physical nature of drug diffusion. For I.V. infusion and certain controlled-release drug products, Ka will be zero-order rate constant.

Ka determined by:

- Method of residuals
- Flip-Flop method of Ka and KE
- Wagner - Nelson Method
- Loo - Riegelman method

## Importance:

Designing a multiple-dosage regimen

Ka and Ke helps to predict peak and trough plasma drug concentrations following multiple dosing.

In bioequivalence studies, drug products are given in chemically equivalent (ie pharmaceutical equivalent) doses. The respective rates of systemic absorption may not differ markedly. For these studies, tmax or time of peak drug concentration can be very useful in comparing the respective rates of absorption of a drug from chemically equivalent drug products.

## Elimination rate constant (Ke):

Ke is summation of rate constants for each process like urinary excretion, metabolism, biliary excretion, pulmonary excretion, etc.

$$KE = Km + Kb + Kl + .......$$

FOR, Zero order rate of elimination is constant irrespective of plasma concentration:

$$Er = KE$$

FOR, First order: Rate of elimination proportional to plasma concentration. Constant Fraction of drug eliminated per unit time.

$$Er = dC/dt = -KE\,C$$

## Importance of elimination rate constant:

- Determination of Ke is important for selection of dose regimen.
- Also in dose adjustment in renal impairment.

## Volume of distribution:

The volume of distribution (VD), also known as apparent volume of distribution, is used to quantify the distribution of a medication between plasma and the rest of the body after oral or parenteral dosing. It is defined as the volume in which the amount of drug would need to be uniformly distributed to produce the observed blood concentration. Volume of distribution may be increased by renal failure (due to fluid retention) and liver failure (due to altered body fluid and plasma protein binding). Conversely it may be decreased in dehydration.

## Equation:

The volume of distribution is given by the following equation

$$VD = \frac{\text{Total amount of drug in body}}{\text{Plasma drug concentration}}$$

## Bioavailability:

The drug, its route of administration and its galenic formulation determine the amount of administered dose absorbed into the circulation. Patient dependant factors also influence bioavailability.

When the drug is administered orally the bioavailability depends on several factors Physicochemical properties of the drug, and its excipients that determine its dissolution in the intestinal lumen and its absorption across the intestinal wall.

1) Decomposition of the drug in the lumen.
2) pH and perfusion of the small intestine,
3) Surface and time available for absorption.
4) Competing reactions in the lumen (for example of the drug with food).
5) Hepatic first-pass effect.

Bioavailability can also be determined for other extravascular routes of administration such as intramuscular, subcutaneous, rectal, mucosal, sublingual, transdermal etc. Sublingual and rectal routes are often used to bypass hepatic first pass effect. Bioavailability of most small molecular weight drugs administered im or s.c. are perfusion rate-limited. Large molecules administered i.m or s.c. enter the blood in part via the lymphatic pathway,

## Renal clearance:

**Definitions:** It is the volume of blood from which the drug is totally removed in unit time through real excretion.

Clearance is the only factor determining the average drug concentration after the iv injection Ma given dose, After an extravascular administration, the average drug exposure is determined both by clearance and by bioavailability. In a multiple dosage regimen, establishing the value of clearance is necessary to predict an average drug concentration within a therapeutic window, The individual factors that can influence clearance are the intrinsic function of liver or kidneys. Therefore, variation of clearance can be anticipated when there is a major impairment of these organs. Blood flow to the organs of elimination can also affect clearance.

Expressed as $CL_R$ it has units: ml/minute

Major Organ for Excretion of Drugs is the Kidney.

Function Units are - Nephron - Bowman's Capsule - Proximal Tubule - Loop of Henle - Distal Tubule - Collecting Duct

$$\text{Renal Clearance (CL)} = \frac{\text{Rate of urinary excretion}}{\text{Plasma drug concentration}}$$

**Physiologically:**

$$\text{Renal Clearance (CL)} = \frac{\text{Rate of filtration} + \text{Rate of secretion} - \text{Rate of reabsorption}}{\text{Plasma drug concentration}}$$

Renal function is determined by measuring GFR, Renal Blood Flow,& Urine flow.

Normal values of: Renal blood flow (RBF) = 1200 ml/min

Glomerular filtration rate (GFR) = 125 ml/min

Urine flow = 1.5 ml/min.

## VIVA-VOCE

**Q.1 Define pharmacokinetics.**

**Ans:** Pharmacokinetics is currently defined as the study of the time course of drug absorption, distribution, metabolism, and excretion. Pharmacokinetics explores what the body does to the drug.

**Q.2 Define pharmacodynamics.**

**Ans:** Pharmacodynamics explores what a drug does to the body

**Q.3 Define biliary excretion.**

**Ans:** Biliary excretion is irreversible transfer of drug or drug metabolites from the plasma to the bile through the hepatocytes (biliary excretion).

**Q.4 Define biological half life.**

**Ans:** The biological half-life or elimination half life of a substance is the time it takes for a substance (drug, radioactive nuclide, or other) to lose half of its pharmacologic, physiologic, or radiologic activity. In a medical context, half-life may also describe the time it takes for the blood plasma concentration of a substance to halve plasma half-life") of its steady-state.

**Q.5 Write down the importance of biological half life.**

**Ans:** Importance of biological half life:

- Adjustment of doses can be made by use of biological half life.
- Dosing regimen can be decided from biological half life.
- It is of very much importance in toxicity studies.

**Q.6 Write down the formula of volume of distribution.**

**Ans:**

$$VD = \frac{\text{Total amount of drug in body}}{\text{Plasma drug concentration}}$$

**Q.7 Define renal clearance.**

**Ans:** Renal clearance is the volume of blood from which the drug is totally removed in unit time through real excretion.

**Q.8 Define bioavailability:**

**Ans:** The drug, its route of administration and its galenic formulation determine the amount of administered dose absorbed into the circulation.

# Experiment No. 15

## Object: To study the biostatistics methods in experimental pharmacology (student's t lest, ANOVA)

## Introduction of Biostatistics:

### Statistics:

It is the science which deals with collection, classification and tabulation of numerical facts as the basis for explanation, description and comparison of phenomenon.

### Biostatistics:

- It is the branch of statistics concerned with mathematical facts and data related to biological events.
- It is the science that helps in managing medical uncertainties.
- Biostatistics covers applications and contributions not only from health, medicines and, nutrition but also from fields such as genetics, biology, epidemiology, and many others.
- It is mainly consists of various steps like generation of hypothesis, collection of data, and application of statistical analysis.
- Any science needs precision for its development.
- Precision is all the more important when it comes to health sciences. For precision; facts, observations or measurements have to be expressed in figures.
- Medicine is essentially an empirical science. It depends on observations and not on theories or theorems.
- As a part of clinical practice or research we deal with many observations, which when systematically arranged, are called Data.
- The process of converting data into information requires a special approach called statistics.
- Statistic' means a measured or counted fact or piece of the information, stated as a figure such as height of one person, birth weight of a baby etc.

## Branches of Biostatistics:

### Descriptive Biostatistics:

Methods of producing quantitative summaries of information in biological science Tabulation and Graphical presentations.

### Inferential Biostatistics:

Methods of making generalizations about a larger group based on information about a sample of that group in biological sciences.

## Primarily performed in two ways:

- Estimation
- Testing of hypothesis

## History:

Sir Francis Galton is considered as the Father of Biostatistics.

He was the first to apply statistical methods to the study of human differences and inheritance of intelligence, and introduced the use of Questionnaires and Surveys for collecting data on human communities, which he needed for genealogical and biographical works and for his anthropometric studies.

## Origin and development of statistic in medical research:

- In 1929, a huge paper on application of statistics was published in physiology journal by Dunn.
- In 1937, 15 articles on statistical methods by Austin Bradford Hill, were published in book form.
- In 1948, a RCT of streptomycin for pulmonary tb., was published in which Bradford Hill has a key influence.
- Then the growth of statistics in Medicine from 1952 was a 8-fold increase by 1982.

## Basis of biostatistics:

### Sources of medical Uncertainties:

- Intrinsic due to biological, environmental and sampling factors.
- Natural variation among methods, observers and instruments etc.
- Errors in measurement or assessment or errors in knowledge.
- Incomplete knowledge.

**Intrinsic variation as a source of medical uncertainties:**

- Biological due to age, gender, heredity, party, height, weight etc. Also due to variation in anatomical, physiological and biomechanical parameters.
- Environment due to nutrition, smoking, pollution, facilities of water and sanitation, road traffic, legislation, stress and strain etc.
- Sampling fluctuations because the entire world cannot be studied and at least future cases can never be included.
- Chance variation due to unknown or complex to comprehend factors.
- Biostatistics is the term used when tools of statistics are applied to the data that is derived from biological sciences such as medicine.
- Any science demands precision for its development, and so does medical science.
- For precision, facts, observations, or measurements have to be expressed in figures.
- Everything in medicine be it research, diagnosis or treatment, depends on counting or measurement.
- High or low blood pressure has no meaning, unless it is expressed in figures
- Thus medical statistics or biostatistics can be called Quantitative medicine.
- In nature, blood pressure, pulse rate, action of a drug or any other measurement or counting varies not only from person to person but also from group to group.
- The extent of this variability in an attribute or a character, whether it is by chance biological or normal, is learnt by studying statistics as a science.
- Variation more than natural limits may be pathological, i.e., abnormal due to the play of certain external factors. Hence biostatistics may also be called a science variation.
- The data after collection, lying in a haphazard mass are of no use, unless they are properly sorted, presented, compared, analyzed and interpreted.
- For such a study of figures, one has to apply certain mathematical techniques called statistical methods.

It is the science which deals with development and application of the most appropriate methods for the:

- ✓ Collection of data.
- ✓ Presentation of the collected data.
- ✓ Analysis and interpretation of the results.
- ✓ Making decisions on the basis of such analysis.
- ✓ Statistics arising out of biological sciences, particularly from the fields of Medicine and Public health.
- ✓ The methods used in dealing with statistics in the fields of medicine, biology and public health for planning, conducting and analyzing data which arise in investigations of these branches.

## Student t Test:

### Introduction:

Biostatistics is contraction of biology and statistics, sometimes referred to as biometry or biometrics, is the application of statistics to a wide range of topics in biology. The science of biostatistics encompasses the design of biological experiments, especially in medicine and agriculture;: the collection, summarization, and analysis of data from those experiments and the interpretation of, and inference from, the results. Hypothesis testing determines the validity of the assumption with a view to choose between two conflicting hypotheses about the value of a population parameter. Hypothesis testing helps to decide on the basis of a sample data, whether a hypothesis about the population is likely to be true or false Statisticians have developed several tests of hypotheses (also known as the tests of significance) for the purpose of testing of hypotheses which can be classified as-

(a) Parametric tests or standard tests of hypotheses
(b) Non-parametric tests or distribution-free test of hypotheses.

Parametric tests usually assume certain properties of the parent population from which we draw samples. Assumptions like observations come from a normal population, sample size is large, assumptions about the population parameters like mean, variance, etc., must hold good before parametric tests can be used. But there are situations when the researcher cannot or does not want to make such assumptions. In such situations we use statistical methods for testing hypotheses which are called non-parametric tests because such tests do not depend on any assumption about the parameters of the parent population. Besides, most non-parametric tests assume only nominal or ordinal data, whereas parametric tests require measurement equivalent to at least an interval scale.

### Use of t-test:

In medical research, t-test is among the three or four most commonly use statistical tests. The purpose of a t-test is to compare the means of a continuous variable in two research samples in orders to determine whether or not the difference between the two observed means exceeds the difference that would be expected by chance from random samples.

Some important terms used in student t-test

### (i) Degree of freedom:

The term degree of freedom refers to the number of observations that are free to vary. The degrees of freedom for any tests are considered to be the total sample size minus 1 degree of freedom for each mean that is calculated. In the student's t-test, 2 degree of freedom are lost because two means are calculated one mean for each group whose means are to be composed. The general formula for the degrees of freedom for the student's two group t-test is N1 + N2 - 2, where N1 is the sample size in the first group and N2 is the sample size in the second group.

## (ii) The t-distribution:

The t-distribution was described by William Goasset, who used the pseudonym "student" when he wrote the description. The normal distribution is the z distribution. The t distribution looks similar to it, except that its tails are somewhat wider and its peak is slightly less high, depending on the sample size. The t-distribution is necessary because when sample size. The t distribution is necessary because when sample sizes are small, the observed estimates of mean and variance are subject to considerable error. The larger the Sample size is the smaller the errors are and the more the t size distribution looks like the normal distribution. In the case of an infinite sample size, the two distributions are identical.

For practical purposes, when the combined sample size of the two groups being compared is larger than 120, the difference between the normal distribution and the t distribution is negligible.

## Technique to perform test:

1. We need to construct a null hypothesis - an expectation - which the experiment was designed to test. For example- If we are analysing the heights of pine trees growing in two different locations, a suitable null hypothesis would be that there is no difference in height between the two locations. The student's t-test will tell us if the data are consistent with this or depart significantly from this expectation. So it is sensible to have a null hypothesis of "no difference" and then to see if the data depart from this.
2. List the data for sample (or treatment) 1.
3. List the data for sample (or treatment) 2.
4. Record the number (n) of replicates for each sample (the number of replicates for sample 1 being termed n1 and the number for sample 2 being termed n2)
5. A significant difference at p= 0.05 means that if the null hypothesis were correct (i.e. the samples or treatments do not differ) then we would expect to get a t value as great as this on less than 5% of occasions So we can be reasonably confident that the samples/ treatments do differ from one another, but we still have nearly a 5% chance of being wrong in reaching this conclusion.

Now compare your calculated t value with tabulated values for higher levels of significance (e.g. $p = 0.01$). These levels tell us the probability of our conclusion being correct. For example, if our calculated t value exceeds the tabulated value for $p = 0.01$, then there is a 99% chance of the means being significantly different (and a 99.9% chance if the calculated t value exceeds the tabulated value for $p = 0.001$). By convention, we say that a difference between means at the 95% level is "significant", a difference at 99% level is "highly significant" and a difference at 99.9% level is "very highly significant".

Statistical tests allow us to make statements with a degree of precision, but cannot actually prove or disprove anything. A significant result at the 95% probability level tells us that our data are good enough to support a conclusion with 95% confidence (but there is a 1 in 20 chance of being wrong). In biological work we accept this level of significance as being reasonable.

Example:

Test workbook (Parametric worksheet: Systolic BP).

Consider 20 first year resident female doctors drawn at random from one area, resting systolic blood pressures measured using an electronic sphygmomanometer were:

| | |
|---|---|
| 128 | 127 |
| 118 | 115 |
| 144 | 142 |
| 133 | 140 |
| 132 | 131 |
| 111 | 132 |
| 149 | 122 |
| 139 | 119 |
| 136 | 129 |
| 126 | 128 |

From previous large studies of women drawn at random from the healthy general public, a resting systolic blood pressure of 120 mm Hg was predicted as the population mean for the relevant age group. To analyse these data in Stats Direct first prepare a workbook column containing the 20 data above or open the test workbook and select the single sample t test from the parametric methods section of the analysis menu. Select the column marked "Systolic BP" when prompted and enter the population mean as 120.

For this example:

Single sample t test

Sample name: Systolic BP

Sample mean = 130.05

Population mean = 120

Sample size n = 20

Sample sd = 9.960316

95% confidence interval for mean difference 5.388429 to 14.711571 df = 19

t = 4.512404

One sided P = .0001

Two sided P = .0002

Power (for 5% significance) = 98.71%

A null hypothesis of no difference between sample and population means has clearly been rejected. Using the 95% CI we expect the mean systolic BP for this population of doctors to be at least 5 mm Hg greater than the age and sex matched general public, lying somewhere between 125 and 135 mm Hg.

## ANOVA:

### Analysis Of Variance (ANOVA):

It is a collection of statistical models and their associated estimation procedures (such as the "variation" among and between groups) used to analyze the differences among group means in a sample. ANOVA was developed by statistician and evolutionary biologist Ronald Fisher. In the ANOVA setting, the observed variance in a particular variable is partitioned into components attributable to different sources of variation. In its simplest form, ANOVA provides a statistical test of whether the population means of several groups are equal, and therefore generalizes the t-test to more than two groups.

**There are two main types**: one-way and two-way.

Two-way tests can be with or without replication.

One-way ANOVA between groups: used when you want to test two groups to see if there's a difference between them.

### Assumptions of ANOVA:

Like so many of our inference procedures, ANOVA has some underlying assumptions which should be in place in order to make the results of calculations completely trustworthy.

They include:

(1) Subjects are chosen via a simple random sample.

(2) Within each group/population, the response variable is normally distributed.

(3) While the population means may be different from one group to the next, the population

Standard deviation is the same for all groups.

Fortunately, ANOVAIS somewhat robust i.e., results remain fairly trustworthy despite mild violations of these assumptions). Assumptions (ii) and (iii) are close enough to being true if, after gathering SRS samples from each group, you:

i. Look at normal quantile plots for each group and, in each case, see that the data points fall close to aline.
ii. Compute the standard deviations for each group sample, and see that the ratio of the largest to the smallest group sample s.d. is no more than two.

## Types of Tests:

There are two main types: one-way and two-way. Two-way tests can be with or without replication.

One-way ANOVA between groups: used when you want to test two groups to see if there's a difference between them.

Two way ANOVA without replication: used when you have one group and you're double-testing that same group. For example, you're testing one set of individuals before and after they take a medication to see if it works or not.

Two way ANOVA with replication: Two groups, and the members of those groups are doing more than one thing. For example, two groups of patients from different hospitals trying two different therapies.

## One Way ANOVA:

A one way ANOVA is used to compare two means from two independent (unrelated) groups using the F-distribution. The null hypothesis for the test is that the two means are equal. Therefore, a significant result means that the two means are unequal.

## When to use a one way ANOVA:

Situation 1: You have a group of individuals randomly split into smaller groups and completing different tasks. For example, you might be studying the effects of tea on weight loss and form three groups: green tea, black tea, and no tea.

Situation 2: Similar to situation 1, but in this case the individuals are split into groups based on an attribute they possess. For example, you might be studying leg strength of people according to weight. You could split participants into weight categories (obese, overweight and normal) and measure their leg strength on a weight machine.

## Limitations of the One Way ANOVA:

A one way ANOVA will tell you that at least two groups were different from each other. But it won't tell you what groups were different. If your test returns a significant f-statistic, you may need to run an ad hoc test (like the Least Significant Difference test) to tell you exactly which groups had a difference in means.

## Two Way ANOVA:

A Two Way ANOVA is an extension of the One Way ANOVA. With a One Way, you have one independent variable affecting a dependent variable. With a Two Way ANOVA, there are two independents. Use a two way ANOVA when you have one measurement variable (i.e. a quantitative variable) and two nominal variables. In other words, if your experiment has a quantitative outcome and you have two categorical explanatory variables, a two way ANOVA is appropriate.

For example, you might want to find out if there is an interaction between income and gender for anxiety level at job interviews. The anxiety level is the outcome, or the variable that can be measured. Gender and Income are the two categorical variables. These categorical variables are also the independent variables, which are called factors in a Two Way ANOVA.

The factors can be split into levels. In the above example, income level could be split into three levels: low, middle and high income. Gender could be split into three levels: male, female, and transgender. Treatment groups are all possible combinations of the factors. In this example there would be 3 x 3 = 9 treatment groups.

## Main Effect and Interaction Effect:

The results from a Two Way ANOVA will calculate a main effect and an interaction effect. The main effect is similar to a One Way ANOVA: each factor's effect is considered separately. With the interaction effect, all factors are considered at the same time. Interaction effects between factors are easier to test if there is more than one observation in each cell, For the above example, multiple stress scores could be entered into cells. If you do enter multiple observations into cells, the number in each cell must be equal.

Two null hypotheses are tested if you are placing one observation in each cell, For this example, those hypotheses would be:

HO1: All the income groups have equal mean stress.

H02: All the gender groups have equal mean stress.

For multiple observations in cells, you would also be testing a third hypothesis:

H03: The factors are independent or the interaction effect does not exist.

An F-statistic is computed for each hypothesis you are testing.

## What is MANOVA:

Analysis of variance (ANOVA) tests for differences between means. MANOVA is just an ANOVA with several dependent variables. It's similar to many other tests and experiments in that it's purpose is to find out if the response variable (i.e. your dependent variable) is changed by manipulating the independent variable., The test helps to answer many research questions, including:

Do changes to the independent variables have statistically significant effects on dependent variables?

What are the interactions among dependent variables?

What are the interactions among independent variables?

## What is Factorial ANOVA:

A factorial ANOVA is an Analysis of Variance test with more than one independent variable, or "factor". It can also refer to more than one Level of Independent Variable, For example, an experiment with a treatment group and a control group has one factor (the treatment) but two levels (the treatment and the control). The terms "two-way" and "three- way" refer to the number of factors or the number of levels in your test. Four-way ANOVA and above are rarely used because the results of the test are complex and difficult to interpret.

A two-way ANOVA has two factors (independent variables) and one dependent variable. For example, time spent studying and prior knowledge are factors that affect how well you do on a test

A three-way ANOVA has three factors (independent variables) and one dependent variable. For example, time spent studying, prior knowledge, and hours of sleep are factors that affect how well you do on a test

Factorial ANOVA is an efficient way of conducting a test. Instead of performing a series of experiments where you test one independent variable against one dependent variable, you can test all independent variables at the same time.

## Variability:

In a one-way ANOVA, variability is due to the differences between groups and the differences within groups. In factorial ANOVA, each level and factor are paired up with each other ("crossed"). This helps you to see what interactions are going on between the levels and factors. If there is an interaction then the differences in one factor depend on the differences in another.

Let's say you were running a two-way ANOVA to test male/female performance on a final exam. The subjects had either had 4, 6, or 8 hours of sleep.

IV1: SEX (Male/Female)

IV2: SLEEP (4/6/8)

DV: Final Exam Score

A two-way factorial ANOVA would help you answer the following questions:

Is sex a main effect? In other words, do men and women differ significantly on their exam performance?

Is sleep a main effect? In other words, do people who have had 4, 6, or 8 hours of sleep differ significantly in their performance?

Is there a significant interaction between factors? In other words, how do hours of sleep and sex interact with regards to exam performance?

Can any differences in sex and exam performance be found in the different levels of sleep?

Example:

| | **Group 1** | **Group 2** | **Group 3** | **Group 4** |
|---|---|---|---|---|
| Sample Size | n1 | n2 | n3 | n4 |
| Sample Mean | s2 | s2 | s3 | s4 |

Four independent groups and a continuous outcome measure. The independent groups might be defined by a particular characteristic of the participants such as BMI (e.g., underweight, normal weight, overweight, obese) or by the investigator (e.g., randomizing Participants to one of four competing treatments, call them A, B, C and D). Suppose that the outcome is systolic blood pressure, and we wish to test whether there is a statistically significant difference in mean systolic blood pressures among the four groups. The sample data are organized as follows: The hypotheses of interest in an ANOVA are as follows:

H0: μ1 = μ2 = p3 ... = μ k

Hl: Means are not all equal.

Where k = the number of independent comparison groups.

In this example, the hypotheses are:

HO: μ1 = μ2 = μ3 = μ4

Hl: The means are not all equal.

The null hypothesis in ANOVA is always that there is no difference in means. The research or alternative hypothesis is always that the means are not all equal and is usually written in words rather than in mathematical symbols. The research hypothesis captures any difference in means and includes, for example, the situation where all four means are unequal, where one is different from the other three, where two are different, and so on. The alternative hypothesis, as shown above, capture all possible situations other than equality of all means specified in the null hypothesis.

## VIVA-VOCE

**Q.1 Define Biostatistics.**

**Ans:** Biostatistics is the science which deals with collection, classification and tabulation of numerical facts as the basis for explanation, description and comparison of phenomenon.

**Q.2 What is ANOVA.**

**Ans:** ANOVA (Analysis of variance) is a collection of statistical models and their associated estimation procedures (such as the "variation" among and between groups) used to analyze the differences among group means in a sample.

**Q.3 Write down the type of ANOVA.**

**Ans:** These are two type:

i. **One-way ANOVA**
ii. **Two-way ANOVA**

# Experiment No. 16

## Object: To study the biostatistics methods in experimental pharmacology (Chi square test, Wilcoxon Signed Rank test).

## Theory:

### Chi Square test:

The primary difference between a chi-square test and the tests we have worked with before is that chi square tests are for used for categorical data. The chi-square test can be used to estimate how closely the distribution of a categorical variable matches an expected distribution (the goodness-of-fit test), or to estimate whether two categorical variables are independent of one another (the test of independence). The chi square test of independence is a natural extension of what we did earlier with contingency tables to examine whether or not two variables appeared to be independent of each other.

In this lesson, we will examine the goodness-of-fit test in more detail.

### Goodness-of-Fit Test

A goodness of fit test is a test that is concerned with the distribution of one categorical variable. The null and alternative hypotheses reflect this focus:

HO: The population distribution of the variable is the same as the proposed distribution

HA: The distributions are different

The Greek letter "chi", written as c, is the symbol used to identify a chi-square statistic, which we will use here to evaluate how well a set of observed categorical data fits a hypothesized distribution. The Chi-Square statistic is actually pretty straight forward to calculate:

$$X^2 = \frac{\Sigma\,(\text{observed - expected})^2}{\text{Expected}}$$

Observed = actual count values in each category

Expected = the predicted (expected) counts in each category if the null hypothesis were true

Conducting a Chi-Square test is much like conducting a Z-test or T-test. We will follow the same basic series of steps and compare a calculated value to a value on a distribution table to evaluate the probability of getting the results we have if the null hypothesis is true, just as we did with the Z and T tests. Now, we will use something called the chi-square distribution table. Additionally, we will be evaluating the number of degrees of freedom, and choosing Values from a chart based on the number. For the goodness-of-fit chi-square test, the degrees of freedom are found by taking, the number of levels in our categorical variable and subtracting one.

## A chi square test will give you a p-value:

The p-value will tell you if your test results are significant or not. In order to perform a chi square test and get the p-value, you need two pieces of information:

Degrees of freedom: That's just the number of categories minus 1.

The alpha level" This is chosen by you, or the researcher. The usual alpha level is 0.05 (5%), but you could also have other levels like 0.01 or 0.10.

**The chi-square distribution** (also called the chi-squared distribution) is a special case of the gamma distribution; A chi square distribution with n degrees of freedom is equal to a gamma distribution with a= n /2 and b 0.5 (or Beta= 2).

## Assumptions of the Chi-Square test

The assumptions of the chi-square test are the same whether we are using the goodness-of-fit or the test-of-independence.

The standard assumptions are:

- Random sample.
- Independent observations for the sample (one observation per subject).
- No expected counts less than five.

Notice that the last two assumptions are concerned with the expected counts, not the raw observed counts.

The chi-squared distribution has many uses in statistics, including:

- Confidence interval estimation for a population standard deviation of a normal distribution from a sample standard deviation.
- Independence of two criteria of classification of qualitative variables.
- Relationships between categorical variables (contingency tables).
- Sample variance study when the underlying distribution is normal.
- Tests of deviations of differences between expected and observed frequencies (one-way tables).
- The chi-square test (a goodness of fit test).

## What does a chi-square test do

Chi-square is used to test hypotheses about the distribution of observations in different categories. The null hypothesis (Ho) is that the observed frequencies are the same as the expected frequencies (except for chance variation), If the observed and expected frequencies are the same, then x' = 0. If the frequencies you observe are different from expected frequencies, the value of x' goes up. The larger the value of y, the more likely it is that the distributions are significantly different.

It is important to note at this point, that that Chi square is a very versatile statistic that crops un in lots of different circumstances. However, for the purposes of this handout we will only concentrate on two applications of it:

**Chi-Square "Goodness of Fit" test:** This is used when you have categorical data for one independent variable, and you want to see whether the distribution of your data is similar or different to that expected (i.e. you want to compare the observed distribution of the categories to a theoretical expected distribution).

**Chi-Square Test of Association between two variables:** This is appropriate to use when you have categorical data for two independent variables, and you want to see if there is an association between them.

## Wilcoxon Signed Rank test:

The Wilcoxon signed-rank test is the nonparametric test equivalent to the dependent t-test.

As the Wilcoxon signed-rank test does not assume normality in the data, it can be used when this assumption has been violated and the use of the dependent t-test is inappropriate. It is used to compare two sets of scores that come from the same participants. This can occur when we wish to investigate any change in scores from one time point to another, or when individuals are subjected to more than one condition.

For example, you could use a Wilcoxon signed-rank test to understand whether there was a difference in smokers' daily cigarette consumption before and after a 6 week hypnotherapy programme (i.e., your dependent variable would be "daily cigarette consumption", and your two related groups would be the cigarette consumption values "before" and "after" the hypnotherapy programme). You could also use a Wilcoxon signed-rank test to understand whether there was a difference in reaction times under two different lighting conditions (i.e., your dependent variable would be "reaction time", measured in milliseconds, and your two related groups would be reaction times in a room using "blue light" versus "red light").

This "quick start" guide shows you how to carry out a Wilcoxon signed-rank test using SPSS Statistics, as well as interpret and report the results from this test. However, before we introduce you to this procedure, you need to understand the different assumptions that your data must meet in order for a Wilcoxon signed-rank test to give you a valid result. We discuss these assumptions next.

## Assumptions:

When you choose to analyse your data using a Wilcoxon signed-rank test, part of the process Involves checking to make sure that the data you want to analyse can actually be analysed using a Wilcoxon signed-rank test. You need to do this because it is only appropriate to use a Wilcoxon signed-rank test if your data "passes" three assumptions that are required for a Wilcoxon signed-rank test to give you a valid result. The first two assumptions relate to your design and the types of variables you measured. The third assumption reflects the nature of your data and is the one assumption you test using SPSS Statistics.

This is another test that is a non-parametric equivalent of a 1-Sample 1-test. The Wilcoxon Signed Rank procedure assumes that the sample we have is randomly taken from population, with a symmetric frequency distribution. The symmetric assumption does not assume normality, simply that there seems to be roughly the same number of values above and below the median. The Wilcoxon procedure computes a test statistic $W_{stat}$ compared to an expected value. $W_{stat}$ that is computed by summing the ranked differences of the deviation of each variable from a hypothesized median above the hypothesized value.

## Example:

The table below shows the hours of relief provided by two analgesic drugs in 12 patients suffering from arthritis. Is there any evidence that one drug provides longer relief than the other.

| Case | Drug A | Drug B | Case | Drug A | Drug B |
|---|---|---|---|---|---|
| 1 | 2.0 | 3.5 | 7 | 14.9 | 16.7 |
| 2 | 3.6 | 5.7 | 8 | 6.6 | 6.0 |
| 3 | 2.6 | 2.9 | 9 | 2.3 | 3.8 |
| 4 | 2.6 | 2.4 | 10 | 2.0 | 4.0 |
| 5 | 7.3 | 9.9 | 11 | 6.8 | 9.1 |
| 6 | 3.4 | 3.3 | 12 | 8.5 | 20.9 |

Solution:

1. In this case our null hypothesis is that the median difference is zero.
2. Our actual differences (Drug B – Drug A) are:

   +1.5, +2.1, +0.3, +0.2, +2.6, -0.1, +1.8, -0.6, +1.5, +2.0, +2.3, +12.4

   Our actual median difference is 1.65 hours.

3. Ranking the differences and affixing a sign to each rank (step 3 and 4 above):

| Diff. | 0.1 | 0.2 | 0 | 0.6 | 1.5 | 1.5 | 1.8 | 2.0 | 2.1 | 2.3 | 2.6 | 12.6 |
|---|---|---|---|---|---|---|---|---|---|---|---|---|
| Rank | 1 | 2 | 3 | 4 | 5 | 6 | 7 | 8 | 9 | 10 | 11 | 12 |
| Sign | - | - | + | - | + | + | + | + | + | + | + | + |

Calculating W+ and W- gives:

$W- = 1 + 2 + 4 = 7\ W+ = 3 + 5.5 + 7 + 8 + 9 + 10 + 11 + 12 = 71$

Therefore, we have n = 12x13

$$\frac{\quad}{2} = 78W = \max(W-,W+) = 71$$

We can use a normal approximation in this case. We have one group of 2 tied ranks, so we must reduce the variance by 8-2

$$\frac{\quad}{48} = 0.125. \text{ We get:}$$

$$Z = \frac{71 - \frac{12x13}{4}}{\frac{\sqrt{12x13x25}}{24} - 0.125} = \frac{71.39}{\sqrt{162.5-0.125}} = 2.511$$

This gives a two sided p-value of p = 0.012. There is strong evidence that Drug B provides more relief than Drug A.

## VIVA-VOCE

**Q.1 Write down the use of Chi square test.**

**Ans:** The chi-square test can be used to estimate how closely the distribution of a categorical variable matches an expected distribution (the goodness-of-fit test), or to estimate whether two categorical variables are independent of one another (the test of independence). The chi square test of independence is a natural extension of what we did earlier with contingency tables to examine whether or not two variables appeared to be independent of each other.

**Q.2 Write down the assumptions of the Chi-square test.**

**Ans:** The assumptions of the chi-square test are the same whether we are using the goodness-of-fit or the test-of-independence.

The standard assumptions are:

- Random sample.
- Independent observations for the sample (one observation per subject).
- No expected counts less than five.

**Q.3 Define Chi-square distribution.**

**Ans:** The chi-square distribution (also called the chi-squared distribution) is a special case of the gamma distribution; A chi square distribution with n degrees of freedom is equal to a gamma distribution with a= n /2 and b 0.5 (or Beta= 2).